The
Complete
Fiber
Fact
Book

The Complete Fiber Fact Book

by
Rita Elkins

Woodland Publishing
Pleasant Grove, UT

Note to Reader: This information is for educational purposes only and is not recommended as a means of diagnosing or treating an illness. All matters concerning physical and mental health should be supervised by a health practitioner knowledgeable in treating that particular condition. Neither the publisher nor author directly or indirectly dispenses medical advice, nor do they prescribe any remedies or assume responsibility for those who choose to treat themselves.

TABLE OF CONTENTS

INTRODUCTION:

THE GREAT FIBER FAMINE

I was raised in an Italian family and most of my fondest recollections are connected to one "food event" or another. Each and every morning my grandmother would begin to prepare the noonday meal, filling the house with tantalizing smells even before my sister and I had left for school. Naturally, what we ate and how we ate it never received much thought. Today, however, in light of what we know about the intrinsic connection of health to diet, I have come to understand the profound value of our childhood eating habits.

Watching my grandmother carefully cook spinach greens, all kinds of legumes including beans, lentils and split peas, enhanced by garlic and onion that had been gingerly sauteed in pure virgin olive oil, the predictable slicing of fresh fruit after each meal, chased by a small glass of chianti, all have scientific significance today. Naturally, my sweet grandmother didn't understand the chemical composition of what she so meticulously prepared, but she did know how to pick high quality fruit and vegetables, insisted on freshness, and even handled food with a kind of respect our microwave dinners have never seen.

In the sixties, when I was preoccupied with mini skirts and fish-net hose, key scientific observations of the Mediterranean diet emerged. Researchers and public health officials noticed that it was unusually health promoting. Detailed analysis of food surveys carried out in Italy allowed a definition of the Italian-style Mediterranean diet to crystalize. Here's how the facts broke down. The diet was:

low in total fat (30 % of energy)
low in saturated fat (olive oil is a monosaturate)
high in complex carbohydrates
high in dietary fiber

I didn't know it at the time but we ate more "plants" than many of my American friend's families, a habit which had health implications far greater than any of us could imagine. Today, media reports reiterate over and over that we need to lower our fat calories, watch out for oils like corn and safflower, and emphasize olive oil, saturated fats, add garlic and onions for their natural immune support, and eat raw fruits and vegetables, and unrefined foods that are still in their whole form. Even the physiologic value of a small glass of red wine to control cholesterol levels has been confirmed in the laboratory. My grandmother's formula was complete.

Unfortunately, as I matured, I found myself falling into more typical American eating habits, switching to white bread, eating more refined, sweet and fatty desserts, skipping the fruit and grabbing a chocolate bar instead. My pantry sported lots of white flour, cooked, canned vegetables, cookies, chips and all those other brightly packaged foods that make you feel like you've "arrived" at food utopia where your family will never be deprived. The foods were virtually "fiberless" and had been so artificially altered from their original state, none of us even knew what they had once been.

So, where did my food choices lead me and my loved ones...to a life plagued with chronic constipation, intestinal gas, bowel disorders, and a whole host of infections. Sounds pretty grim doesn't it...where was my grandmother when I needed her?

The cold hard facts are that we, as a society are suffering from a deplorable lack of fiber in our diets..a fiber famine, if you will. Yes, we are constantly assaulted with reports, news flashes, medical articles and scientific statistics warning us that diets low in fiber can literally kill us...yet we persist to eat the way we always have, usually turning up our noses at anything too brown or too green and making the mistake of believing that our daily bowl of wheaties is more than fiber adequate. We need to wake up and pay attention to facts such as:

- Dietary fiber intake can decrease our sensitivity to insulin and raise blood sugar, in addition, eating foods that are whole and full of nutrients effects the rise of blood sugar the least. (This explains why a bowl of Captain Crunch for breakfast can send you on a blood sugar roller coaster).

- THE MORE FIBER YOU EAT, THE MORE FAVORABLE YOUR CHOLESTEROL LEVELS WILL BE.

- CERTAIN FIBER SUPPLEMENTS CAN ACTUALLY SUPPRESS THE INCIDENCE OF COLON CANCER.

- THE LIGNIN FIBER CONTENT OF SOME PLANTS CAN INHIBIT CERTAIN BAD ESTROGENS WHICH HAVE BEEN LINKED WITH BREAST CANCER

- THE TRANSIT TIME OF DIGESTED FOOD IN THE GASTROINTESTINAL TRACT IS DECREASED WITH A HIGH FIBER DIET, FACILITATING THE REMOVAL OF TOXIC SUBSTANCES, RADIOACTIVITY AND DAMAGING HORMONES.
- FIBER REDUCES THE ABSORPTION OF FAT BY DRAWING WATER INTO THE INTESTINAL

SYSTEM AND CREATES A SENSATION OF FULLNESS WITH LESS CALORIC INTAKE.

• WHEN NUTRITIOUS, HIGH FIBER DIETS ARE CONSUMED, FOOD CRAVINGS DIMINISH.

These facts concerning fiber only reveal the tip of the iceberg. Fiber is full of remarkable surprises and applications.

You'd think with this kind of information at our fingertips, we'd do a little "pantry cleaning" and cook more like my grandmother. To the contrary, many of our children are raised on foods that are deplorably low in roughage. The price we all pay is that they routinely become constipated at an early age. Moreover, all kinds of health problems that don't even seem remotely connected to eating fiber can develop, and we often lament that our kids are always sick.

A 1995 clinical study found that the dietary fiber intake of children has remained the same over the last 12 years, which has been well below the recommended level.[1] What this study also found was that if we feed our children high fiber diets, they will consume less fat, particularly saturated fats.

Sadly, we pay more attention to keeping our cars running well than our own digestive systems. The bottom line (no pun intended) is that fiber keeps our human machinery running smoothly. Preventing the build-up of any kind of waste material is crucial to the maintenance of any machine. If the fuel filter in your car is clogged, your engine is going to spit and sputter and your gas milage will be significantly reduced. You can spend a small fortune on fancy gasoline and carburetor additives, but until you replace that filter, your car will run poorly.

Likewise, the human machine becomes terribly sluggish if its systems are not efficiently cleared of toxic waste. To make matters worse, all of our body systems, not just the digestive are affected and compromised. So, why do we consume such horribly high amounts of caffeine, white sugar, white flour, alcohol and gobs of meat?

In our body-image obsessed society, why do we spend millions of dollars trying to lose weight on all kind of crazy diets when we know that cultures that routinely eat high fiber diets have a very low incidence of obesity? Unquestionably, these people don't count calories to maintain their weights.

Today, we know the facts. We can't claim ignorance to justify our food choices. FIBER CAN SIGNIFICANTLY DETER POTENTIALLY FATAL DISEASES, CONTRIBUTE TO WEIGHT CONTROL AND PROFOUNDLY IMPROVE OUR HEALTH AND WELL BEING. OK, we know that now, so why do we continue to spite ourselves by grabbing the sweet role rather than the apple? The issue of convenience and availability of certain foods comes into play here. We may even have to put ourselves out a bit to be healthy.

Our bodies are trying to tell us something. Italians are trying to tell us something. Dietary profiles of Italy have confirmed that eating Mediterranean style can lower blood lipids, and protect against carcinogens and free radicals. How plant components affect our health has become increasingly important in understanding the make-up of chronic and degenerative diseases. The question for us is...are we listening?

FIBER— FACT OR FICTION:
FIND OUT IF YOU'RE A FIBER FLUNKIE

Before we begin our excursion through the wonderful world of fiber, take a minute and quiz yourself. If you're like me, you'll be surprised at how little we really know about this marvelous food component. Each correct answer is worth one point. Make sure to total your score and grade yourself accordingly.

TRUE OR FALSE FIBER QUIZ

1. Fiber is another name for bran.

2. All fiber, regardless of its source, essentially affects the body in the same way.

3. Tougher cuts of beef have more fiber than tender cuts.

4. Peeling and juicing fruits actually increases their fiber content.

5. Cooked vegetables and fruits have less fiber than raw ones.

6. Eating bran or wheat germ is just as nutritious as eating the whole grain these foods were isolated from.

7. Carrots contain more total fiber than potatoes.

8. Eating a bowl of cooked Cream of Wheat supplies more total dietary fiber than a bowl of Lucky Charms.

9. One reason you should not overeat fiber rich foods is that you will become nutrient deficient.

10. You can gain weight just as easily from eating too many whole apples as you can from drinking their juice equivalents because the calorie content is the same.

11. Fiber passes through the small intestine unchanged but is always digested in the large intestine.

12. Eating white bread that has been fortified with all the vitamins and minerals we need is as nutritious as eating a slice of whole wheat bread.

13. Having a lettuce salad with plenty of tomatoes and cucumbers everyday is a good way to fill our fiber requirements.

14. If we eat three, well balanced meals per day we shouldn't need a fiber supplement.

15. Substituting unbleached flour for bleached flour increases its fiber content.

FOR THE CORRECT ANSWERS, REFER TO PAGE 187.

CHAPTER ONE

FIBER VINDICATED

I always find it rather amusing to see all the fuss the medical establishment makes over a health-promoting discovery which natural health advocates have been preaching for decades. So it is with fiber. Champions of whole grain, raw foods have been rightfully corroborated by experts who now enthusiastically nod their heads in favor of fiber. Fiber has become a buzz word of the nineties. Recently, or maybe a better term should be "finally" the American Medical Association joined the National Cancer Institute, the American Heart Association and the American Dietetic Association in urging us, (the general public) to eat adequate amounts of whole-grain foods, legumes, and fruits and vegetables.

You might say that fiber has finally been vindicated in the late 20th century, however, its historical evolution reaches far back into the days of ancient medicine. As usual, what we assume is a modern, new health revelation had its roots in antiquity.

A TWENTIETH-CENTURY TRAGEDY

Hippocrates, the Father of Medicine highly recommended eating whole wheat "for its salutary effects upon the bowels." Roman athletes took this advice seriously and ate whole grains believing that their endurance and strength would be preserved. Despite his approval of whole wheat, even Hippocrates believed that more refined flours were superior because bowel movements were smaller and that must be good. Wrong.

Since these very early days, whole grains were typically consumed, especially by lower class societies who could not afford the fatty, sweet, high protein diets of their king's table. Unfortunately, progress took a substantial step backwards when the medical view of fiber was literally reversed in the 18th and 19th centuries. Low-fiber, white, wheat flour was hailed as a more available and economical source. Fine sieve roller milling brought white flour home to every table, and the fiber famine commenced.

Interestingly, certain health advocates in our country protested this view and vigorously tried to promote the merits of bran to the American public. Up until this period of time, fiber had comprised a great part of our diets. Now, fiber-free foods such as white bread and sugar were seen as signs of affluence and progress. Dr. J. H. Kellogg, who was none the less still impressed with the value of whole grains, introduced toasted wheat flakes to the nation's breakfast tables in 1895.

Unfortunately, the high grinding system of milling spread quickly to Western countries and resulted in a dramatic decrease of cereal consumption and a rise in sugar and fats. Today we eat only around a fifth of the whole grain cereal we used to..a practice which started our day with a substantial dose of fiber. No more.

It's no coincidence that as our intake of fiber decreased, certain bowel disease such as colon cancer and diverticulosis increased. Ironically, physicians of the late 19th and early 20th centuries prescribed the worse possible treatment for these bowel disorders: eating a bland, highly refined diet! To put things into perspective, there are over 85,000 cases of colon cancer diagnosed in our country annually and the number is growing.

In the early 20th century, the science of fiber actually began, the term "fiber" was coined and studies were initiated. Subsequent subjects included the laxative action of bran which was immediately rejected by the American Medical Association; consequently, the publications ceased.

In 1953, cereal shortages in Great Britain made it necessary to mill high fiber flour and substances like cellulose, and lignin were analyzed and determined to be very relevant to human nutrition. In 1947, despite what some physicians were telling their patients, bran was not found to be a gastrointestinal irritant. A man named Walker had the audacity to confront the medical establishment by stating that dietary fiber may protect against specific disorders including: constipation, appendicitis, diabetes, gallstones, obesity and coronary heart disease.[2] Folks, that was almost fifty years ago!

In the sixties, researchers noticed that certain diseases that ravaged our societies were relatively rare in third-world communities. Obviously, affluence is not always a good thing. Surgeon General T.L. Cleave even went as far as to say that all the diseases of civilization were caused by the "saccharine disease." refering to our blatant over-consumption of sugar and refined carbohydrates.[3]

The seventies gave us reports like that of Dr. Burkitt's work in Uganda. He discovered that eating high levels of dietary fiber increased the frequency of bowel movements and the size of the stool as well. He found that rural South African blacks had about one-half the stool transit time and over double the stool weight of affluent blacks or whites.

Not surprisingly, the medical community was slow to catch on to what these findings implied. Official articles on fiber in reputable medical publications were a rare occurrence. The role of dietary fiber was typically brushed off by many health practitioners. The question here might be, "what does it take to get their attention?"

Fortunately, today, the medical establishment has become more fiber aware, however, unlike the lone voices of the past that tried to extol the virtues of "roughage," they are slow to speak out and even slower to prescribe. We have Cleave, Campbell and Burkitt to thank for their tireless efforts in promoting the consumption of fiber. By so doing, they had to suffer the indignities reserved for proponents of medical quackery.

THE NUTRITIONAL REVOLUTION

The incredible role that fiber plays in our total nutrition was emphasized by Donald McLaren in 1988. He claimed that three revolutions in nutrition had taken place in recent history (thank goodness).

1. THAT SOME DISEASES CAN RESULT FROM A VITAMIN DEFICIENT DIET.

2. THAT GOOD NUTRITION DOESN'T JUST INVOLVE PREVENTING A DEFICIENCY BUT IS BASED ON AVOIDING AN EXCESSIVE INTAKE OF CERTAIN THINGS LIKE FAT, SALT AND WHITE SUGAR.

3. THAT CONSUMING ADEQUATE AMOUNTS OF DIETARY FIBER CAN HAVE A PROFOUND EFFECT ON THE MAINTENANCE OF OUR HEALTH.[4]

What a change in attitude from the casual brushing off of diet and nutrition as nothing less than trivial factors in controlling disease and safeguarding our health.

A PALEOLITHIC PERSPECTIVE ON FIBER: WE HAVEN'T PROGRESSED MUCH

Experts tell us that at least 65% of paleolithic diets were comprised of fiber. Just to bring home how fiber deficient we are, our diets have less than half this amount. While our constitutions and genetic make-ups are still basically the same as they were 40,000 years ago, our nutrition is not. In our case, progress has backfired on us taking us a giant step backward in providing modern food processing techniques that routinely take the fiber out of the food. How our ancient ancestors ate is very relevant to us today, as we enter a new millennia. Just looking at the amounts of key fiber foods we consumed in the eighties as compared to 1910, and 1930 in pounds, charts our so called "progress" in this area.

FOOD	1910	1930	1984
FRUIT	176 LBS	199 LBS	143 LBS
POTATOES	205 LBS	147 LBS	90 LBS
FLOUR & CEREAL	291 LBS	204 LBS	135 LBS5

REFINED FOODS: AN INSULT TO MOTHER NATURE

Eating overly processed, fatty, sweet foods have become the rule rather than the exception in American families. Much of the food we consume today has been fragmented, chemically altered and unnaturally preserved. In addition, we're now eating non-food substitutes as if they were the real thing. Aspartane, saccharine, fake fats, artificial textures, colors, etc. get casually popped into our mouths with no real thought given to their long term effects. Most of us assume if the FDA says something is OK to eat, then it is. Michael Jacobson in the April, 1975 edition of *Smithsonian* states:

> The United States, not surprisingly, has been the leader in the genetic engineering of food crops and in the laboratory creation of new foods. Benjamin Franklin and Abraham Lincoln, if they could visit us, would probably have some difficulty distinguishing between a toy store and a supermarket. They would not even recognize as foods such products as artificial whipped cream in its pressurized can, or some breakfast "cereals" that are almost half sugar and bear little resemblance to cereal grains...Many of the new foods do save us time and trouble, but they are often costly, in terms of both dollars and, ultimately, health.

The sad fact is that most of us don't eat well, much less get enough fiber. How many of us gulp down a bowl of sugary cereal or a sweet roll for breakfast, wash it down with one or more cups of coffee, have a caffeine drink and cheese tortilla for lunch and then order a pepperoni pizza for dinner? Our love affair with creamed

soups, puddings, ice cream, gravies, sugary gelatin, white flour pastries like doughnuts, noodles, enormous quantities of meat and gallons of pop has taken an enormous toll on our health and is innately linked to the frightening escalation of cancer and degenerative diseases. All of these foods are virtually fiber free. Many of us have been guilty of teaching our kids to turn up their noses at any food that is brown, textured, or speckled.

Dr. Oscar Janiger M.D. in his book *A Different Kind of Healing* referring to a physician who was interested in the healing properties of foods and plants states:

> "His interest in the healing properties of foods and plants, he said, dates back to the Great Depression, when he was fed whole grains and helped his family grow organic vegetables: `It taught me where foods come from. My parents would take white bread and roll it into a ball and bounce it off the floor saying, this is not food for humans.'"

Some of our children and some of us, for that matter, would not even recognize certain foods in their whole, unchanged states. For the most part, whole foods that come from the plant kingdom offer us significant dietary fiber. While food producers and manufacturers have been adding natural and synthetic fibers to foods, they cannot improve on Mother Nature's creations.

"Many of us have only vague notions about what our food was like in its fresh and natural state. Between the fresh, natural, whole food and its refined fractionate commercial product there is an abyss of lost nourishment, even when the refined food has been enriched."[6]

In the short space of one year, the average American eats:

100 lbs. of refined sugar
55 lbs. of fats and oils
300 cans of soda pop
200 sticks of gum
63 dozen doughnuts
50 lbs. of cakes and biscuits
20 gallons of ice cream
18 lbs. of sweets and candy
5 lbs. of potato chips
7 lbs. of corn chips, popcorn and pretzels[7]

WE'VE BEEN THROWING THE BABY OUT WITH THE BATHWATER

In our attempt to make food more visually appealing, digestible, whiter etc. we have routinely separated and discarded some of the fiber fractions of food as they are supplied by nature. We have a modern fetish for trying to improve on food, as if Mother Nature's version of food was just to too crude or primeval for our refined tastes. We remove grain polishings from rice, de-wheat germ and de-chaff wheat, eat the potato and throw out the peel, and cut the crusts off of already bleached white bread. Removing the fiber from agricultural products has traditionally occurred to create greater consumer appeal.

"Thus, wheat flour, with the bran removed, could produce a very white bread with a soft, easy-to-chew cohesive texture. Without the bran fiber present, salivary enzymes could work more quickly on the starch of the bread, to release glucose, giving the bread made from

refined flour a sweeter taste than its coarser, fiber-filled counterpart, which was made from whole wheat flour."[9]

TAMPERING WITH WHOLE FOODS HAS EXACTED AN ENORMOUS TOLL

We've got to start making the connection with what we casually put in our mouths and how we feel today and will feel tomorrow. Mother Nature knew what she was doing in providing humankind with whole and complete foods that should not be tampered with. Isn't it a paradox that when it came to fiber the smarter we got, the less nutritious our diets became.

Smashing, stripping, and squashing whole foods inevitably depletes them of their natural fiber content. So many of our foods have been artificially manipulated. Eating foods as nature meant them to be is almost unheard of today. Just walk down the aisles of any "super" market. You'll be horrified to find than most of the foods we buy in cans or brightly colored packages rarely resemble "real foods." To make matters worse, most of us have never even thought of checking for fiber content. We need to repent.

OK, so now that we've got a pretty clear picture what sophisticated food processing has done to fiber, let's be precise about the true, technical definition of fiber. While we see fiber currently hyped in our magazines and newspapers and have experienced the see-saw mentality toward oat bran mania, we need to learn the facts so we don't fall prey to marketing strategies.

THE ABSOLUTE SUPERIORITY OF WHOLE, UNFRAGMENTED FOODS

Much of the information in this book regarding fiber suggests using wheat or oat bran. While the advantages of bran cannot be disputed, it is only one part of the whole grain as mother nature created it. Ideally, if we stocked our kitchens with whole wheat, millet, barley, whole oats etc., we wouldn't need to buy grain isolates like bran to get our colons up to snuff.

So much of the research we have on fiber has been done on grain fragments such as bran and not on the whole grain. Eating whole grain intact and in its entirety has not received the scientific attention it requires. Concerning dietary fiber, we must understand that its physical form determines how it will behave in the intestines. It's time to concentrate on the value of whole foods rather than their separate nutrients.

Like medicinal plants, whole grains have been intrinsically designed with a wide array of inherent components which potentiate and complement each other. Like isolating pharmaceutical agents from herbs to create synthetic drugs which have various bad side effects, separating grain constituents may not be as desireable as eating the whole food, the way nature intended. Annmarie Colbin, in her book *Foods and Healing* writes:

"..instead of eating a vegetable in the shape in which it grows, we consume it in fragmented form, its separate components split apart, we are not following the natural scheme of things. When we consume wheat germ, white flour and bran separately, it is not the same as eating them in their natural, integrated and properly balanced state as whole wheat....a hundred or so years ago,

CHAPTER TWO:

LOW FIBER DIETS: THE DISASTROUS CONSEQUENCES

Diets that lack fiber allow the food we consume to remain in the intestines longer. In fact, bland, refined diets such a white flour breads, pies, pastries etc. can actually stick to our colon walls and may never be properly eliminated, causing all kinds of bowel problems.

When food waste stays in the colon and is not quickly expedited through the bowel, toxins can build up. This toxin component has been linked to the development of several seemingly unrelated diseases. Naturally, colon disorders such as colitis and colon cancer are involved. Fiber boosts waste through the intestinal canal to be expelled within a reasonable time from consumption.

Direct results of highly refined, low fiber diets include chronic constipation and hemorrhoids. Low fiber foods such as white flour products and mushy, overly cooked foods don't have the boosting and bulking power of whole grains and raw fruits and vegetables.

THE CONCEPT OF WESTERN DISEASES

More changes have occurred to what we eat and how we eat it in the last 200 years than in the last 2000. Interestingly, while we continue to prosper economically and continually advance technically, our nutritional habits place us behind certain third-world countries.

What's happened is that we have replaced fiber-rich foods with elevated consumption of salt, fat, animal protein and sugar. Consequently, we have to deal with a whole array of diseases which are relatively rare in third-world countries. Consider the following quote from Denis Burkitt:

> "I was able to collect, with the assistance of various agencies from over 600 third-world hospitals, information regarding the rarity of such common diseases in the west as gallstones, colon cancer, diabetes, coronary heart disease and varicose veins; and to obtain from more major medical institutions evidence on the virtual absence of diverticular disease of the colon and hiatus hernia."[10]

FIBER DEFICIENT DIETS CAN RESULT IN THE FOLLOWING PHYSIOLOGICAL CHANGES:

* a decrease in bowel movements
* a longer transit time
* changes in stool consistency (less formed)
* increase in constipation

NOT EATING ENOUGH FIBER CAN LEAD TO:

APPENDICITIS
COLITIS
COLON CANCER
CONSTIPATION
CORONARY HEART DISEASE
CROHN'S DISEASE
DIVERTICULITIS
GALLBLADDER DISEASE
GALLSTONES
HYPERLIPIDEMIA (High Cholesterol Levels)
ILEITIS
IRRITABLE BOWEL SYNDROME
DIABETES (LATE ONSET)
OBESITY
VARICOSE VEINS[11]

If you can believe it, the above list comprises a conservative estimate of disorders that can develop if we keep eating the way most of us are eating. Current studies have also linked low fiber diets with other kinds of cancer as well. Because fiber helps to scoot toxic substances our of our bodies, hormonally linked diseases may also be affected. For women, in particular, bad forms of estrogen can stay in the body longer if waste material sits in the bowel too long.

So, the cold hard facts tell us that despite the many health benefits of fiber, Americans are still eating fiber deficient diets. The average daily intake of fiber is between 11 and 13 grams, far below the recommended 35 grams.[12]

CHAPTER THREE:

OUR BOWELS ARE TRYING TO TELL US SOMETHING

The fact that almost half the world is constipated conveys a very clear and simple message...whatever it is that we're eating or not eating, our colon's are not happy. The human machine is marvelously designed to function efficiently. It can take in food, begin to chemically breakdown the chemical structures of that food through chewing and salivary enzymes, continue digestion in the stomach, absorb nutrients for fuel and regeneration in the small intestine, move waste to the large intestine and in a relatively short amount of time, should expel that waste from the body.

This is the way we were meant to operate. Unfortunately, many if not most of us don't. To make things even worse, few of us are aware of the profound health implications of conditions like constipation. Medical practitioners rarely emphasize the very vital role that our bowel plays in determining how we feel, whether we get sick or even the likelihood of our premature deaths. Have you ever heard of the term "transit time?" I never had, but believe me, it will be an integral part of my vocabulary from now on.

TRANSIT TIME

Transit time simple refers to how long it takes for something that you eat to travel from your mouth, through your stomach and small intestine to your colon. As mentioned early, western nations that eat diets low in fiber have longer transit times than third-world countries. It's commonplace for an American to have a transit time of three days to two weeks in cases of severe constipation. Eight to 35 hours is typically seen in cultures where whole grains, fruits and plants are routinely consumed.

Normally, adults who eat from 35 to 45 grams of fiber every day have an average transit time of approximately 36 to 48 hours. Transit time can vary from person to person, and if you're a woman, it can be 24 % slower than for men. Changes in transit time from one day to the next are also common, however, it's not normal to have three bowel movements a day and than go without one for a week.

You can test your transit time by eating beets, taking two tablespoons of liquid chlorophyll, or ingesting charcoal tablets which can be purchased at your pharmacy. Record when you ate the beets or took the tablets and watch for either the purple or the black to show up after a bowel movement. Ideally, the trip should take less than 36 hours. If it takes longer, look at your diet and beef up on fiber.

Increasing the fiber content of your diet is the one most important thing you can do to decrease your transit time. Dr. James Scala, in his book, *Eating Right for a Bad Gut*, writes:

"Adding guar gum to food increased the transit time by 75 minutes, pectin by 15 minutes, and cellulose had no effect. This tells us that the largest amount of time that food spends in our body is its residence in the large intestine. But it also tells us that passage through the small intestine is influenced by fiber..."

Doing something as simple as adding bran to your meals can have a dramatic effect on transit time.

"The transit time was shortest with bran, vegetables and fruit in this order and was more highly correlated with fecal form than other bowel function measurements. Contrary to popular thinking, there was no association of transit time with age: both young and old subjects had faster transit times (a difference of half a day) than those aged 14-45 years.[13]

WHY WORRY ABOUT TRANSIT TIME?

The longer waste material stays trapped in the colon, the greater the risk of various potentially harmful situations.

1. Toxic compounds are created when putrefaction occurs. These compounds can find their way back into the bloodstream, where the liver has to filter them out again. Some of these chemicals are carcinogenic in nature. This process is referred to as auto-intoxication by some health care practitioners. Some of these harmful compounds include:

   bile salts
   volatile fatty acids
   heavy metals
   pigments and preservatives
   toxins which include: phenol, cadaverian, butyric acid, botulin, putrescin, ammonia, creosole, and sepsin[14]

2. Long transit times are usually associated with poorly formed stool that lacks water. People who have to strain to have a bowel movement put additional pressure on the intestines and may be prone to developing hemorrhoids and diverticula.

3. Long transit times can result in chronic intestinal gas and even in diarrhea, which is actually a form of constipation in some cases.

FECAL INDICATORS

As indelicate a subject as it is, the size and consistency of the stool is a good indicator of fiber intake. When you lack fiber you may have scant, dry bowel movements that require a great deal of straining to excrete. Pressure which results from these difficult bowel movements can cause veins in the anus to swell and form painful hemorrhoids. Remember what fiber advocates found in Africa...high fiber diets produced sizeable, soft stool that was frequently eliminated. Clearly, a correlation exists between stool weight and health. Observing our solid waste can tell us a great deal about our state of health.

Having a bowel movement should not be a dreaded event or occur sporadically. Our country spends more on over-the-counter laxatives than any other country on earth. Are we clueless? The problem is clearly a lack of fiber and can be easily and economically remedied. Our white bread, meat and potato diets don't deliver.

****FIBER TIDBIT****
It takes fifty loaves of white bread to provide our ideal daily fiber intake of 35-40 grams.

CHAPTER FOUR:

WHAT IS FIBER?

Fiber has been called roughage and is technically a food component that remains undigested as it is processed through the gastrointestinal tract. Because it readily absorbs water, it helps to form the bulk required to create a good ol fashioned bowel movement. Having a colon that functions well has a profound impact on all of our other body systems. The word fiber is easily misunderstood and applies to a number of substances.

TECHNICALLY SPEAKING.....Fiber is a complex carbohydrate consisting of a polysaccharide and a lignin substance that gives structure to the cell of a plant. It is the portion of plant food which is not digested. Insoluble fiber has the ability to pass through the intestines intact and virtually unchanged. Unlike fats, carbohydrates and proteins, fiber does not provide the body with nutrients or fuel for energy. It usually has no caloric value.

Dietary fiber is found only in plant components such as vegetables, fruits and whole grains. There are primarily two types of fiber; soluble and insoluble. Some foods contain both types:

Soluble Fiber: Fiber eventually digested in the large intestine, so its bulking power is limited. Soluble fibers can dissolve in water have been linked to the following actions:

- help prevent blood sugar highs and lows
- lower blood cholesterol
- lower the risk of heart disease
- help to control high blood pressure
- encourage friendly bacteria to grow

Insoluble Fiber: Fiber, which for the most part, remains undigested and promotes a faster stool transit time.

Insoluble fibers can:

* keep the bowel clean and operative and helps bind dangerous toxins and hormones for better excretion
* fosters regularity
* contributes to better digestion
* prevent constipation
* helps lower the risk of bowel disease

SOURCES OF SOLUBLE FIBER

Soluble fiber is found in pectin, lignin, gums and mucilages and includes: psyllium, beans, apples, pears, oat bran, etc. This type of fiber usually doesn't fit our notion of fiber. It is digestible, and when broken down, it creates a kind of gel as it absorbs water in the intestinal tract. Unlike insoluble fiber, this type does not bulk the stool to the extent of insoluble fiber, but it does have a tendency to slow down the rate at which food is digested.

Pectin, gums and mucilage are all soluble fibers and are discussed in a later section. Soluble fiber is found in vegetables, particularly onions, bulbs, leeks and asparagus, Fruit, including dried varieties are soluble fibers. Interestingly the insoluble fiber content of fruits is found in its flesh and stringy membranes rather than its peelings.

SOURCES OF INSOLUBLE FIBER

This type of fiber is primarily composed of cellulose and hemicellulose. Cellulose is a non-digestible form of fiber which is present in the outer portions of vegetable and fruits. It is usually found in their crunchy, woody, stems, stalks, and peels. In addition, the bran or seed covering of whole grains is another type of insoluble fiber. Hemicellulose fibers have the ability to remain unchanged and absorb water as they travel through the digestive tract. They increase stool bulk and transit time which prevents constipation and conditions like hemorrhoids. Stalks, stems, peels and fruit and vegetable skins are all made up of insoluble fiber.

TOTAL DIETARY FIBER

This term refers to the sum of the soluble and insoluble fiber content of a particular food. We need a good variety of foods that contributes to at least 35 grams of fiber to our diet each and every day. Most foods contain both types of fiber. Unfortunately the foods which are the most fiber rich are rarely housed in our pantries.

Few families wake up to whole grain cereal, a consistent supply of raw fruits and vegetables and the continual consumption of legumes like split peas, beans, lentils or whole grains like millet and barley. Statistics reveal that most of us get 9 grams of fiber per day if we're lucky...a statistic that has to change if we plan to live a long and healthy life.

GENERAL PROPERTIES OF FIBER

• IT HOLDS ON TO WATER

Insoluble fiber like bran contains fancy sounding sugars called hydrophilic polysaccharides which swell up and create a viscous gel in the small intestine when then combine with water. Pectins, gums, and mucilages have a high affinity for water so they make excellent laxative and bulking agents. This ability to hold water and form gels increases intestinal transit time and adds weight and substance to the stool.

• FIBER AND FERMENTATION

Virtually all dietary fiber enters the intestine in an unchanged form. The presence of fiber encourages bacterial fermentation during the digestive process. For example, pectin is completely metabolized in the intestines, whereas wheat bran is not. The digestibility of fiber depends on:

a. its chemical structure
b. the amount of friendly bacterial flora present
c. the length of time it stays in the intestines (transit time)

Metabolizing fiber in our bodies is an anaerobic process and one of the products of this process is gas.

• THE ABSORPTION ABILITY OF FIBER

Dietary fiber has the wonderful ability to soak up various deleterious substances we could well do without. Fiber can absorb:

drugs
toxic chemicals
bile salts
hormonal components

FUNCTIONS OF FIBER IN A NUTSHELL

Fiber has to be the single most important factor in maintaining the health of the gastrointestinal tract, not to mention its protective role against several potentially fatal diseases. Eating fiber rich foods can prevent and treat disease. WHY? Let's look into exactly what eating fiber does in the human body.

FIBER HAS THE ABILITY TO:

- increase fecal bulk by retaining water
    psyllium
    wheat bran
    rice bran

- decrease stool transit time
    psyllium
    pectin
    wheat bran

- keep blood sugar levels more stable
    guar gum
    pectin
    oat bran
    tragacanth gum

- lower blood serum and liver cholesterol (lipids)
    psyllium
    oat bran
    guar gum
    pectin

- help prevent weight gain by slowing the rate of digestion and absorption and helps to control hunger

- expedite the removal of potentially dangerous toxins and carcinogens from the bowel by acting as a carrier and by boosting elimination.

- bind with bile salts which can help decrease the risk of gallbladder disease and certain types of cancer.

- create the presence of healthier intestinal bacteria.

CHAPTER FIVE

KINDS OF FIBER

The notion that fiber is fiber is fiber is not true. All fibers are not created equal. We hear so much hype about the value of different kinds of fibers and their advantages, we may feel that we need to be a biochemist to decipher a food label. Technically, there are seven forms of fiber, each with its own specific function.

1. PECTINS:

Pectin slows the absorption of food after meals, and is recommended for anyone with hypoglycemia or diabetes because it causes blood glucose levels to rise more gradually. I routinely use pectin when I make homemade preserves for its thickening property. Pectin also has the ability to help remove toxins and metals, reduces blood cholesterol levels, and reduces the risk of heart disease and gallstones. Pectin becomes water soluble in ripened fruit. Pectins can also bind bile acids which helps us keep our gallbladders healthy.

SOURCES: carrots, beets, cabbage, citrus fruits, apples, grapes, bananas, cabbage, okra, dried peas, green beans, onion skin, and sugar beet pulp.

2. CELLULOSE:

This insoluble source of fiber is a carbohydrate which is the main structural component of the outer covering of vegetables and fruits. It is the fibrous part of the cell walls of these plants. It helps to nourish the blood vessels so it is beneficial for varicose veins, colitis, constipation and hemorrhoids. Cellulose has also proven its ability to rid the colon of carcinogenic substances. It also has the ability to significantly increase fecal weight. It can bind up water very impressively. Make sure to check what kind of cellulose you may be getting when you buy certain food items. Wood pulp can be added to foods to increase their fiber intake. While this type of cellulose is permitted on a very limited basis, we all need to know if we're eating wood pulp.

SOURCES: wheat bran, beets, peas, broccoli, carrots, lima beans, pears, apples, Brazil nuts, whole grains and green beans.

3. HEMICELLULOSE:

Like cellulose, hemicellulose is not digestible and is considered a complex carbohydrate. It comprises the matrix of the cell walls of plants, which are filled with cellulose fibers. This type of cellulose is chemically broken down through the action of certain friendly bacteria in the bowel and can cause gas in some individuals. Hemicellulose has a remarkable ability to retain water. It is recommended for weight loss, colon cancer, constipation and for removing cancer causing substances which can inhabit the bowel.

SOURCES: psyllium seeds, oat bran, apples, pears, bananas, beans, corn, cabbage, whole grains, peppers, and green vegetables.

EXAMPLE OF HEMICELLULOSE: PSYLLIUM SEED

Psyllium is a hemicellulose and has traditionally been called the "mother of herbs" in ancient Anglo-Saxon poetry. Psyllium is a hardy, roadside botanical whose seed husk is an excellent intestinal cleaner and stool softener. Today, psyllium has practically become a household word, and is commonly used in several over-the-counter laxatives. Psyllium thickens very quickly. Anyone who has mixed up a glass of Metamucil knows how quickly it must be consumed before it solidifies.

Psyllium seeds are covered with mucilage, which we have just discussed. Because mucilage swells when it comes in contact with water, it works to bulk up the stool and promotes movements of the bowel. It can also help to soothe inflamed tissue and promote the growth of friendly bacteria. The value of psyllium in keeping blood cholesterol levels down has recently been confirmed. Even the American Heart Association recommends adding psyllium to our diets for its cholesterol-lowering properties.[15]

Most of us are probably unaware that psyllium can keep our blood sugar levels more stable. More detail on the effects of fiber on hypoglycemia and diabetes is offered in a later chapter. Familiar laxatives which use psyllium include:

Metamucil™
Correctol™
Fiberall™

It's important to know that many natural health advocates would recommend using natural laxatives like psyllium that don't contain artificial colors or metals like aluminum.

The typical dose of psyllium is one to two rounded teaspoons in a full glass of water taken after a meal. Psyllium is safe for children and can be taken consistently. Psyllium seed is one of those botanical wonders which provides human beings with an invaluable service. Psyllium gently boosts the colon with little or no side effects.

WATCHWORD: Many of the psyllium products sold in the United States have been diluted with rice hulls.

4. LIGNIN:

Lignins are a non-carbohydrate cell wall material that are made up of chemical polymers and aromatic alcohols. Lignin contributes to the rigidity of plant cell walls and inhibits cell wall digestion by intestinal bacteria. Lignin has shown its ability to help lower blood serum cholesterol levels and to prevent the formation of gallstones. It does this by binding with bile acids which can ultimately contribute to the formation of stones. It is also transformed by intestinal bacteria into a type of lignin which helps inhibit the action of bad estrogens, which have been linked to the development of breast cancer. Lignin is recommended for anyone with diabetes, breast, or colon cancer.

SOURCES: flaxseeds, wheat, potatoes, apple, cabbage, peaches, tomatoes, strawberries, Brazil nuts, carrots, peas and green beans.

EXAMPLE OF LIGNIN FIBER: FLAXSEED

Flaxseeds contain essential fatty acids and lignin. Essential fatty acids have been strongly linked to keeping the cardiovascular system healthy and contributing to thermogenesis or fat burning. Essential fatty acids can not be synthesized by the body and must be ingested. Flaxseed are rich in the Omega-3 factors and in magnesium, potassium, vitamin D and E, B-vitamins, amino acids and fiber.

Supplying the body with essential fatty acids from flaxseed can help achieve balanced weight loss. It is believed that flaxseed oil can actually simulate brown fat stores in the body to burn more fat. Consider the following quote:

"Omega-3 fatty acids can actually increase metabolic rate. They also rid the body of excess fluids and can increase energy levels. The best source of Omega-3 fatty acids is organic flaxseed oil."[16]

Because flaxseed is a lignin fiber, it can act as an anti-carcinogenic, an anti-estrogenic and as an antioxidant in the body.

5. GUMS:

Gums are complex polysaccharides that are water soluble. Their role in plants is to repair damaged areas. Various gums are used in the food industry. The following list below will be familiar to many of us, who, up until now, may have been quite miffed by these exotic sounding ingredients. With the ever increasing popularity of fat free foods that have a gooey, creamy texture, gums and mucilages are experiencing a new renaissance.

EXAMPLES:

- **Guar gum (guar flour):** Comes from a plant which is native to India and is tasteless, odorless and completely water soluble. It serves as a protective colloid, a thickener and is primarily used in very thick viscous liquids or spreadable foods.
- **Gum Arabic:** This gum comes from the Acacia tree and consists of a variety of sugars. It is commonly used to maintain food product flavor and long shelf-life.
- **Flaxseed Gum:** Used as a substitute for Gum Arabic, this gum is used in similar applications. The whole flaxseed is sometimes added to cereals for its laxative action.
- **Karaya Gum (Indian Tragacanth):** A white, slightly acidic gum with a mild acidy odor, Karaya serves as a texturizer, thickener and food emulsifier.
- **Locust Seed Gum (Carob Flour):** This gum swells in cold water and goes clear in hot. It has a legume-like flavor and serves as a binder and thickeners. It has been used as a substitute for cocoa, chocolate and coffee.
- **Psyllium Seed Gum:** Psyllium seeds are one of the best natural laxative promoters. As a gum, it has a very high level of soluble dietary fiber and is added to some cereal products for this reason.
- **Xanthin Gum:** Usually sold as a potassium salt, Xanthin Gum is a microbial gum. It serves to form a film, has good heat resistance and can stabilize and thicken food products.

Most of these gums are extruded from the stems or seeds of tropical or sub-tropical trees and shrubs. Gums can form gels in the small intestine and also help to bind acid and other organic waste material.

6. MUCILAGES:

Mucilages are routinely obtained from seeds and seaweeds and are used as thickening and stabilizing agents like gums. They effectively hold water and can serve as excellent bulking agents.

SOURCES: legumes, psyllium, guar

EXAMPLES:

- **Agar:** A sweet mucilage that can remain stable in high temperatures and is often used for thickening dairy products and confections.
- **Alginate:** Extracted from brown seaweed, it gives foods a creamy texture and inhibits the formation of ice crystals. This is one of those "mystery" ingredients we often see on ice cream cartons.
- **Carrageenan:** Another seaweed mucilage which is typically used to gel and emulsify certain foods.

BRAN FIBERS

The word *bran* refers to the fibrous covering which surrounds certain whole grains. Bran is technically referred to as a cereal fiber and is the portion of the grain which was discarded from whole wheat as waste when modern milling processes were established at the turn of the century. Bran has excellent stool bulking capacities and can significantly reduce transit time. To a great degree, bran was no longer consumed after the introduction of refined flours. It's no coincidence that as bran consumption dwindled, the incidence of certain so called "western" diseases escalated.

Bran has the ability to hold water better than any other source of fiber. Different cereal brans have their own individual chemical construction and so their ability to retain water can vary.

FIBER TIDBIT

Bran and Guar Gum are effective fiber sources for increasing fecal weight.[17]

OAT BRAN

Over the last decade, oat bran has enjoyed a high level of publicity, some good, some not so good. When original scientific findings on the benefits of oat bran hit the media, a veritable oat bran frenzy resulted. Oat bran mania was born, and for a time, it was looked at as a health panacea. While eating oat bran may not get rid of cellulite, it can help to lower blood cholesterol, thereby preventing heart disease.

Technically, oat bran is made by grinding the inner husk of the whole oat grain. Study after study has confirmed that consistently eating oat bran can lower high blood serum cholesterol as much as 20 percent or more. Even already low blood cholesterol can be reduced by 5 percent by consuming daily doses of oat bran. It is the soluble fiber found in oat bran that makes is an impressive fiber source.

Before we all run out and buy oat bran, it must be understood that oat bran must be eaten consistently and indefinitely to maintain its ability to lower cholesterol. In addition, having a bowl of hot oat cereal and then eating a diet that is high in animal fats is not recommended. Oat bran can only do so much and cannot undo the harm of a diet that is loaded with saturated fats. In order for oat bran to work its magic, it should be combined with a diet that is low in animal fats and rich in fruits and vegetables.

Remember that oatmeal, which is the ground version of the whole oat grain contains about one third less fiber than the bran.

WATCHWORD: Be careful not confuse the term "oat fiber" for "oat bran." Oat fiber additions to certain commercial products may originate from oat hulls which is a type of insoluble fiber.

SAMPLING OF THE OAT BRAN CONTENT OF CEREAL PRODUCTS

Quaker: Mother's Oat Bran
   2/3 Cup Cooked ....28 Grams

Quaker: Oat Bran Ready To Eat Cereal
   3/4 Cup...20 Grams

Health Valley: Oat Bran Flakes
   1/2 Cup...15 Grams

Nabisco: Wholesome and Hearty Oat Bran
   1/3 Cup...14 Grams

Kellogg: Common Sense Oat Bran
   1/2 Cup...13 Grams

Ralston Purina: Oat Bran Options
   1 Cup..10 Grams

General Mills: Cheerios
1 1/4 Cups ....8 Grams

Post: Honey Bunches of Oats
2/3 Cup.......................................1 Gram

MUFFINS

Healthy Valley Oat Bran Fancy Fruit
  Raisin Muffin ....17 Grams

Pepperidge Farm Oat Bran with Apples
  Muffin ....9 Grams

Lender's Oat Bran Bagel ....7 Grams*

**taken from a chart prepared by Gail Zyla, M.S., R.D.

Keep in mind that oat bran is not the only kind of fiber that lowers blood serum cholesterol levels. Legumes, which refers to all kind of dried beans, psyllium, carrots and pectin, can also lower cholesterol levels.

WHEAT BRAN

Wheat bran has excellent stool bulking capacities and has been used therapeutically to lower blood sugar and blood cholesterol levels. It helps to "sweep' out the intestinal tract of potentially dangerous chemical compounds including carcinogens which can induce the formation of tumors. When you buy a box of unprocessed bran, it is usually of the wheat variety. Wheat bran is comprised largely of insoluble cellulose and hemicellulose fibers.

While adding bran to beef-up the fiber content of foods is desireable, obtaining bran in its natural state, as part of the whole wheat grain is preferable. Anytime the original state of a food is altered, some of its nutritive value will be compromised. If you find it difficult to eat foods in their whole grain state, then adding bran to meatloaf, casseroles, breads and cereals is highly recommended. The best way to eat foods, however, is in their whole state, the way Mother Nature intended.

FIBER TIDBIT

Cooking wheat bran actually alters it so that is has less effect on the intestinal tract than raw bran. If you want optimal transit speed, look for wheat bran that is unprocessed and in its raw form.

BARLEY BRAN

Barley is relatively untapped as a wonderful source of fiber and other valuable nutrients. Studies have shown that barley fiber can lower both serum and bile cholesterol levels, inhibiting the formation of gallstones. The chemical constituents of barley bran resemble oat bran and have been shown to also protect against the development of certain types of cancer.

The darker the barley grain is, the more nutritious it is thought to be. Barley juice has been used for generations to treat gastrointestinal disorders and helps to heal irritated intestinal tissue.

Certain antioxidant compounds have recently been identified in barley bran which look very promising. Using whole or ground barley in soups and cereals is not only delicious, but extremely nutritious as well.

RICE BRAN

Rice bran, like barley bran contains some very desireable chemical constituents. Rice bran oil contains oryzanol which can lower cholesterol levels and discourage the accumulation of arterial plaque (only brown rice, not white varieties contain these compounds).

Again, the desirability of eating whole, brown rice has to be stressed. Very few of us cook with brown rice and have even resorted to minute rice, which must be fortified to have any nutritive value. The complex, synergistic effects of eating rice in its original state cannot be overstated. Like all the other grains we've talked about, processing brown rice so that it loses its bran covering has profound health implications. Rice bran is high in vitamin B and contains a number of other nutrients. White rice is fattening and lacks these nutrients (not a good trade off).

Fiber Tidbit

Rice bran when combined with fish oil can help to boost thermogenesis (fat metabolism) and may help to explain why certain cultures who subsist on brown rice and fish have an extremely low incidence of obesity.

FRUIT AND VEGETABLE FIBERS

Fruits supply a source of fiber called pectin. Apple pectin has been used to help control cholesterol levels and stabilize blood sugar. The pectin content of fruits like apples and pears has the ability to increase the time food stays in the stomach, which is a good thing. Gastric-emptying is the first phase of the transit of waste material from the stomach to the colon. Citrus peels are also used as a source of pectin.

NOTE: Some laxatives contain pectin, which is derived from citrus peelings.

Studies have been conducted to determine other beneficial attributes of fruit pectin. Some of these include:

- Pectin can help protect us against potentially harmful food additives and other toxins which we inadvertently consume on a regular basis.
- Pectin can help to enhance our ability to metabolize glucose
- Pectin may have the ability to lower plasma-cholesterol levels
- Research suggests that pectin may act as an immune stimulant, boosting the natural defenses systems of the body.

APPLE PECTIN

Apple pectin has already demonstrated its ability to raise blood sugar levels more slowly than fruits like grapes, honeydews, strawberries or oranges.[18] When insulin-dependent diabetics took apple pectin as a supplement before eating a meal, they required significantly less insulin to return their blood sugars to normal.[19] In addition, taking therapeutic doses of apple pectin may lower blood serum cholesterol levels.

Consistently eating fresh, raw, apples and pears is certainly recommended as a great way to add pectin fiber to your diet. If you don't like apples or pears, you can purchase apple pectin in supplement form. Vegetable fibers found in beets and carrots are excellent sources of both soluble and insoluble fiber.

BEET FIBER

Beets are rich in vitamin B6 and should ideally be eaten in their raw state. The fiber content of beets is impressive, to say the least. While beet fiber may not be as easy to purchase as apple pectin is, it is becoming more available through health food stores. Again, eating the food in its natural, whole state is always preferable to altered forms.

Beet fiber has been associated with the following physiological actions: the improvement of glucose tolerance the lowering of serum cholesterol levels, the normalizing of blood pressure, and the enhancement of zinc and iron absorption.[20]

FIBER TIDBIT
Gram per gram, beet fiber has more soluble and insoluble fiber than oat bran.

CARROT FIBER

Carrot fiber, like beet and pectin fruits has also been associated with its ability to control cholesterol levels. It helps to bind bile salts, which we know are related to cholesterol levels and the development of gallbladder disease. Carrots should be eaten raw and should be consumed liberally on a regular basis. Remember that while drinking carrot juice may have its nutrient value, eating the whole carrot supplies more fiber and less calories.

CHAPTER SIX

CONQUERING FIBER PHOBIAS

How many of us were raised to turn up our nose at green foods, brown coarse foods or stringy vegetables? Granted, changing eating habits ingrained in us from childhood is not an easy task. While most of us would like to go on believing that our low fiber diets are perfectly healthy, the facts cannot be denied. It may sound a bit radical, but many of us exist on foods which can literally act like poisons in our bodies.

Our poor dietary habits (too much fat, sugar, salt, meat and lack of fiber) are directly linked to the worst fatal diseases we face as a society. Now that's enough to make us get phobic. Getting back to good old fashioned nutritious eating may be hard, but it's certainly attainable. The key is to start slowly and to gradually change the way we and our families eat.

HOW MUCH FIBER DO WE NEED?

A good diet should include 25 to 35 grams of fiber or at least 1 ounce of dietary fiber each and very day. Some health practitioners are recommending up to 50 grams of fiber per day. Two thirds of that fiber should be insoluble. Adding wheat bran to your diet is the easiest way to boost your fiber intake. The average American eats from 9 to 13 grams of fiber per day. The ideal barometer to determine if you're getting enough fiber is whether you have a good bowel movement at least every 24 hours. Your transit time is also very important. Unless you suffer from certain bowel conditions like Crohn's disease or ulcerative colitis, some experts believe that you can't get too much fiber.

WATCHWORD: Make sure you're not hypersensitive or allergic to grain and certain high fiber legumes. An intolerance to gluten can result in gas, diarrhea, and abdominal cramping which can result in celiac disease and malabsorption of nutrients. Find out what forms of fiber agree with you if you are food sensitive.

CAN YOU GET TOO MUCH FIBER?

While this subject spawns considerable debate, some health care experts believe that eating more than thirty-five grams of fiber per day may adversely affect vitamin and mineral absorption. While this is technically true, it is rarely the case because most of us eat nowhere near the amount of fiber we need. Cultures that routinely eat 60 grams of fiber per day are not necessarily vitamin or mineral depleted and can be considered well-nourished.

While it is true that some fibers may absorb calcium, zinc, iron and magnesium and that the presence of fiber in the intestines may inhibit the absorption of certain nutrients, these effects are present only under extreme conditions.[21] In other words, don't let the fear of becoming nutrient deficient stop you from boosting you fiber intake. This particular phenomenon does not pose a significant threat. The marvelous benefits of fiber far outweigh the very remote possibility that you will eat quantities large enough to pose any problem.

WATER AND FIBER GO TOGETHER

Remember that eating more fiber means drinking more water. Because fiber absorbs water like a sponge, if you don't drink enough, you may have some intestinal distress. A lack of water can result in bowel movements that are difficult to pass. Stool that is high in fiber and low in water can become hard and dry, defeating fiber's primary purpose. Drinking plenty of pure water is good for weight maintenance, supple skin and healthy kidneys. If you do increase your fiber intake, you'll probably experience increased thirst. Listen to your thirst receptors and drink, drink, drink.

HOW TO BECOME FIBER-FRIENDLY

Alright...we're ready, we're convinced and we want to repent of our fiberless ways, but we're not sure how to do it and still enjoy eating! So let's start at the beginning with what some people have called the most important meal of the day; breakfast. If you don't want to eat a hot steaming bowl of whole wheat cereal or oatmeal, make or buy high quality whole grain breads and create a meal out of toast and fresh fruit. Cereals that have good fiber content include: Bran Buds, All-Bran, Bran Flakes, and Oat Bran.

Because it's difficult to calculate exactly how much dietary fiber a particular food supplies, the best way to approach diet is to eat plenty of raw fruits and vegetables with their skins left on. Use unprocessed or minimally processed grains and cereals. Dried peas, beans, lentils etc. are excellent sources of fiber and are low fat to boot. Nuts and seeds like pumpkin, sunflower and sesame are good fiber sources, but also contain significant amounts of fat.

Virtually any inclusion of beans (navy, pinto, kidney), or grain bread in the diet can significantly increase fiber levels toward recommended amounts. If you don't have time to cook beans (it's really just a matter of putting them on in the morning, that's all) then use canned, pre-cooked beans and add them to anything and everything.

****FIBER TIDBIT****

Did you know that a half-cup serving of pinto beans supplies four grams of fiber.

GETTING USED TO A HIGH FIBER DIET

If you've been used to eating processed, refined low fiber foods and you switch to a high fiber diet, you may experience cramping, bloating diarrhea and gas. Ironically, even constipation can occur if you neglect to drink inadequate amounts of water. The operative term here is "moderation." Start slowly with cereals like wheat bran or beans and gradually increase your intake. If you do this, your intestinal tract will adjust nicely and you'll be less "gassy."

FIBER FLATULENCE

You see, when you eat fibrous foods, bacteria in the bowel attack and digest these complex carbohydrate molecules and in the process methane gas is released. This is the "bean" effect so many of us are familiar with. Individual reaction to fiber will greatly vary from person to person. The intestinal bacteria responsible for these side effects will gradually adjust to the increased fiber load. Any unpleasant symptoms should decrease and eventually disappear.

Make sure to eat slowly and chew well. Digestive enzymes that break down carbohydrates must be initially activated in the saliva. This can only happen if the food remains in the mouth long enough and is properly broken down by the teeth. Anyone who is used to "snarfing" their food will probably tell you that gas is a problem. Sending large quantities of poorly chewed food to the stomach has already increased your gastric workload. Be kind to your intestinal tract by chewing your food well.

Lastly, watch what gives you gas and eat less of it.

NOTE: Some people believe that taking supplemental digestive enzymes right before eating can cut down on the formation of gas.

REMEMBER TO:

• Add fiber gradually
• Drink plenty of water
• Chew your foods thoroughly so that the necessary digestive enzymes to to digest the food will be activated in the saliva

SIMPLE AND PAINLESS WAYS TO INCREASE YOUR FIBER INTAKE

• Take a good fiber supplement every morning with your breakfast or 30 minutes before any meal.
• Grab a handful of oat cereal when you get the urge to snack.
• Add bran, millet, barley etc. to your meatloaves, casseroles, pancakes, cake and cookie batters, stuffings, and compotes.
• Use crunchy granola cereals or barley nuts as a topping for ice cream, yogurt, baked potatoes, fish,

salads, etc. Adding whole wheat that has been soaked to salads is delicious. Always add seed or fresh raw fruit to make yogurt more fiber acceptable, and only buy active culture yogurts.

- Eat fresh, raw fruit and vegetables with their peelings whenever possible.
- Reach for prunes, dates, or figs when you need to appease your sweet tooth instead of cookies, candies or juice.
- Look for fiber-rich foods offered in salad bars and add them liberally (broccoli, carrots, red beans, garbanzo beans, sunflower seeds etc.).
- Get in the habit of sprouting your own legumes. Peas, lentils, mung beans, garbanzo beans, lentils, soybeans, wheat, etc. can all be sprouted and make delicious additions to tossed green salads.
- Buy canned, pre-cooked beans of all kinds and add them to salads, soups, casseroles and stews.
- Keep a good supply of grains on hand that you can add to any recipe to make it more nutritious and "fibery." Good grains are millet, barley, brown rice, whole oats and whole wheat.

CHAPTER SEVEN:

FOODS AND THEIR FIBER VALUE

You may think that it sounds rather boring to have to eat plenty of apples, beans or any other single fiber rich food everyday. Think again. Generously consuming a variety of vegetables and fruits is vital to a number of highly developed cuisines. Italian and Japanese dishes routinely use whole grains, vegetables legumes and fruits in a delicious assortment of easy-to-fix dishes. Fruit is a food type that most of us rarely get enough of and should be the object of our food cravings for something sweet.

Fresh, raw, whole fruits and vegetables may appear to have a poor fiber showing per 100 grams, however, they have marvelous nutritive properties and should ideally be combined with whole grain cereals. Don't try to eat just one kind of fiber. Fiber is what gives fruits and vegetable their structure and solidity.

It is for this very reason that eating whole fruits and vegetables is much healthier for us than drinking their juice. While these juices are full of nutrients, frequently their fiber content has been removed. For this reason, the way in which fruit glucose enters our bloodstream will be altered. If we eat a whole apple or orange, we get the sugar combined with the fiber. It will move into the bloodstream at a slower rate and be digested differently.

If you're sugar sensitive, don't drink fruit juices which can dramatically shoot up your glucose levels. Eat the whole fruit with its peeling whenever possible. The difference between the way we assimilate whole fruits and fruit juice has nothing to do with calorie content.

FIBER TIDBIT
Eating fruits and vegetables in their original, unaltered state can produce different physiological effects than mashing, juicing or peeling them.

THE CASE FOR BEANS

The nutrient composition of legumes, like dry beans, makes them the perfect food prescription for good health. Eating beans increases our consumption of starches and complex carbohydrates and can satisfy hunger without copious amounts of fat. Dry beans supply the human body with protein, fiber and essential vitamins and minerals. They are naturally low in fat and sodium and contain no cholesterol.

The marvelous health benefits of beans have been documented over and over. Eating more beans is a superb way to increase dietary fiber. Look over the recipes found in the back of this book and incorporate more beans into your meals.

FOODS WHICH CONTAIN NO FIBER

dairy products (milk, cheese, yogurt, sour cream, buttermilk etc.), animal meats

FOODS WITH A RELATIVELY LOW FIBER CONTENT

leafy vegetables (lettuce, cabbage, watercress, etc), some fruits

FOODS WITH A MODERATE FIBER CONTENT

root vegetables (beets, turnips, carrots, potatoes, parsnips, yams)

FOODS THAT ARE HIGH IN FIBER

legumes (split peas, dried beans, lentils), seeds, nuts and dried fruits (especially figs, dates and prunes).

FOODS WITH THE HIGHEST FIBER CONTENT

whole grains (wheat, oats, millet, rice, corn, barley and buckwheat)

TOTAL FIBER BREAKDOWN OF FRUITS AND VEGETABLES FROM HIGH TO LOW IN GRAMS

FRUITS	SERVING	SOLUBLE	INSOLUBLE	TOTAL
RASPBERRIES	3/4 C.	.37	6.43	6.80
PEAR	1 (med.)	1.00	4.00	6.00
APPLE	1	.84	1.96	2.80
BANANA	1 (med.)	.64	1.36	2.00
ORANGE	1 (sm.)	.88	.88	1.20

VEGETABLES				
ASPARAGUS	3/4 C.	.81	2.29	3.10
CARROTS	1/2 C.	1.11	1.19	2.30
BROCCOLI	1/2 C.	.88	1.12	2.00

POTATO	1/2 (med.)	.95	.95	1.90
TOMATO	1/2 C.	.20	.60	.80
LETTUCE	1/2 C.	.13	.17	.30

**adapted from a chart prepared for *New Facts About Fiber.*

Can you see why eating a lettuce salad everyday is not a good source of dietary fiber. Salad bars are great, however, they do not usually provide enough dietary fiber. Adding garbanzo or kidney beans, corn, whole wheat, broccoli, carrots, and beets can raise the fiber value of your salad. Learn to spot fiber friendly veggies and add them liberally. Remember that just because a vegetable looks stringy or "fibery" doesn't mean that it is.

FOOLHARDY FIBER SOURCES

Several misconceptions exist about certain foods that are thought to be high in fiber but aren't. One of the most common ones is the notion that if you eat a lot of lettuce salads, you're getting plenty of fiber. Lettuce, tomatoes and even celery are not considered excellent sources of fiber. They are, in fact, much lower in fiber than legumes and whole grains. So, while these veggies provide some fiber, by themselves they are an insufficient source.

WATCH OUT FOR TERMS, NAMES OR APPEARANCES WHICH YOU MAY ASSUME ARE SIGNS OF HIGH FIBER FOODS. SOME OF THESE INCLUDE:

- Brown colored breads, rolls, cookies etc. caramel coloring is frequently added to food products to make them appear more appealing or natural.

- Terms such as: Wheat, wheatberry, multigrain, natural, fortified, etc. none of these means that the whole grain has been used. Many products with these kinds of names are mostly comprised of white flour. Even the term "Whole Wheat" doesn't necessarily mean that all of the flour used has been milled from the whole grain.

- Watch our for naughty, high fat baked good which are disguised as fiber rich foods. Oat-bran doughnuts, cookies or even tortilla chips are commonly high in fat and sugar and notoriously low in oat bran. A New York Times survey showed that some "Oat Bran" muffins contain so little oat bran that they are virtually useless as a source of fiber.

- A single bran muffin can contain as much fat as 3 lunch size bags of potato chips. Just because it has bran in it, doesn't necessarily make it good for you. The use of coconut oil, hydrogenated vegetable fats, linseed oil etc. have all been linked to coronary artery disease.

- New varieties of snack crackers that sound fibery are really nothing but doctored up white flour foods. Many whole grain saltines, wheat crackers etc. fall into this category. Always check for fiber content and ingredient listing.

- Nuts can be a good source of fiber but they usually come salted, processed and are often rancid. Look for raw nuts, preferably unshelled such as almonds, pistachios etc.

- Just because something is crunchy or requires chewing doesn't mean it has a high fiber content. Celery is one of those tough vegetables that is all crunch and low fiber.

HOW TO CHOOSE A GOOD BREAD

It's so easy to think that you're buying high fiber bread if it appears brown, or has a "fibery" sounding name. The terms "wheatberry" "wheat" bread or "multigrain" do not always mean that the bread is a good source of fiber. Unfortunately, fiber content on bread labels is rare. So, look for whole grain or whole wheat as the first ingredient listed on the label. Rye bread consists of white flour that has been "peppered" with isolated grains of rye and is essentially the same as white bread. Sourdough bread does not contain more fiber than regular white bread. Sprouted-grain breads can be quite nutritious and are marvelous substitutes for anyone who might be allergic to wheat.

NOTE: The new, nifty all-in-one bread makers that grind, mix and bake bread all in the same unit are fun and provide a wonderful way to have a warm, homebaked loaf of whole wheat bread waiting for you when you get home.

COOKED FRUITS AND VEGETABLES CAN BE FIBER ALTERED

The canning process which places fruits and vegetables in a boiling water bath can break down and alter the fiber content of these foods, not to mention destroying some very valuable nutrients as well. Try to avoid processed foods and reach for the raw fruit or vegetable. In this way, you get all kinds of fiber in its natural proportionate mix as nature intended. Some foods like millet and potatoes have to be cooked in order to "pop" open their fiber components.

FOOD FIBER CONTENT CHARTS AND TABLES

The following tables list certain food groups and their total fiber content in grams. Look over the list carefully. Its findings may surprise you. I was shocked that certain foods I had been eating which I assumed to be much more fibrous than others were, in fact, lower in fiber. This also brings home the fact that just because a food is brown, doesn't mean it has a lot of fiber value.

Look over all the tables and remember that our goal is to design daily menus with foods that will give us at 35 to 40 grams of fiber per day. Most of these figures came from the Nutrient Data Group of the Department of Agriculture.

COMPARISON OF THE FIBER CONTENT OF SOME FOODS*

FULL FIBER	FIBER DEPLETED	FIBER FREE
WHOLE WHEAT BREAD	BROWN BREAD	SUGAR
BROWN RICE	WHITE BREAD	VEGETABLE OIL
ROLLED OATS	WHITE RICE	HONEY
PEANUTS	ORANGE JUICE	WINE
EDIBLE DRY BEANS	APPLESAUCE	BEER
FRESH VEGETABLES	TAPIOCA	SYRUPS
FRESH FRUIT	MOST COLD CEREALS	MILK CIDER

*adapted from a chart prepared for *Handbook of Dietary Fiber*

COLD CEREAL FIBER COUNTS

- 12 GRAMS OF FIBER PER SERVING:

General Mills Fiber One
Kellogg's All Bran Extra Fiber

- 9 GRAMS OF FIBER PER SERVING

Nabisco 100% Bran
Kellogg's All Bran

- 3 TO 5 GRAMS OF FIBER PER SERVING

Post Natural Raisin Bran
Post Bran Flakes
Post Fruit N' Fiber

General Mills Raisin Nut Bran

Kellogg's Bran Flakes
Kellogg's Cracklin Oat Bran
Kellogg's Raisin Bran

Ralston Bran Chex

Quaker Corn Bran

Nabisco Shredded Wheat
Nabisco Oat Bran

CEREALS WITH LOW OR NO FIBER COUNTS

General Mills
100% Natural

Crispy Wheat
Crunch Berries

Trix
Instant Oatmeal

Cocoa Puffs

Lucky Charms
Cheerios

Wheaties
Honey Grahamm
Corn Chex

Rice Chex
Wheat Chex
Product 19
Dinosaurs
Just Right

Apple Jacks
Nuggets

Nut & Honey Crunch
Cocoa Pebbles
Corn Flakes
Smurf Magic Berries
Rice Krispies
Super Golden Crisp

Frosted Flakes

Croonchy Stars

Cream of Wheat

Shocked? I was. This table made me look at the slogan, "Trix is for kids" in a whole new light. Notice how many of the heavily advertised sugary cereals that target our children are low in fiber. Now, while the fiber content of certain cold cereals may seem adequate, they may also contain too much sugar or fat. Read your labels carefully and don't sacrifice one nutrient for another.

FRUIT

When choosing fruit, keep in mind that those with edible skins and those with seeds usually have the highest fiber contents. Whole, raw apples and pears are excellent and readily available high fiber fruits. Look over the following chart and make sure to notice how much lower the fiber content of juiced fruit is than the whole version.

FRUIT	FIBER IN GRAMS
Apple (1 medium)	3.2
Apple Juice (1/2 C	.4
Applesauce (1/2 C)	2.1
Apricots (3 medium)	2.1
Avocados (1/2 average)	1.6
Bananas (1 medium)	3.0
Blackberries (1/2 C)	4.5
Blueberries (1/2 C)	3.0
Cantaloupe (1/2 medium)	1/6
Cherries (10)	.9
Dates (4 pitted)	3.2
Grapes (1/2 C)	.5
Grapejuice (1/2 C)	.6
Grapefruit (1/2 medium)	1.1
Grapefruit Juice (1/2 C)	trace
Honeydew (small wedge)	1.5
Kiwi (1 medium)	3.4
Orange (1 medium)	2.8
Orange Juice (1/2 C)	.6
Papaya (1 medium)	1.8
Pears (1 medium)	4.0
Pineapple (1 slice)	1.5

Plums (3 medium)	1.8
Prunes (1.2 C pitted)	2.4
Raisins (1/4 C)	2.5
Raspberries (1/2 C)	9.2
Strawberries (1/2 C)	1.5

VEGETABLES

Edible skinned vegetables with seeds, like fruit, are also good fiber choices. Look over the following chart and you'll probably be surprised again. Crunchy vegetables like celery, carrots and cucumbers are lower in fiber than spinach and squash.

VEGETABLES	FIBER IN GRAMS
Asparagus (4 spears)	1.3
Beans, (green 1/2 C)	2.1
Beans (wax) (1/2 C)	2.1
Beets (diced 1/2 C)	1.4
Broccoli (1/2 C)	3.8
Brussels sprouts (1/2 C)	2.3
Cabbage (1/2 C shredded)	2.1
Carrots (1 medium)	1.5
Cauliflower (1/2 C)	1.1
Celery (3 stalks)	1.5
Coleslaw (1/2 C)	.8
Corn (1/2 C)	4.7
Cucumber (1 medium)	1.7
Eggplant (1/2 C)	2.5
Lettuce (1/2 head)	.3
Mushrooms (1/2 C)	.8
Okra (1/2 C)	1.6
Onions (1.2 C)	1.6
Peas (1/2 C)	5.7
Peppers (1/2 C)	1.0
Potatoes	
baked (1 medium)	2.6
mashed (1/2 C)	2.5
french fried (10)	2.6
Radishes (4 small)	1.3

Rutabagas (1/2 C)	1.7
Sauerkraut (1/2 C)	2.1
Spinach (1/2 C)	6.5
Squash	
Acorn (1/2 C)	6.0
Zucchini (1/2 C)	2.0
Sweet Potatoes (1 small)	3.7
Tomatoes (1 medium)	1.8
Turnip Greens (1/2 C)	1.6
Turnips (1/2 C)	1.0

BEANS AND LEGUMES

This is one food group that we don't take full advantage of. Protein-rich beans and other legumes like split peas and lentils are superb sources of fiber. By contrast, animal sources of protein that we just can't seem to get enough of (meat, poultry, fish, eggs, and dairy products) contain no fiber whatsoever.

BEANS AND LEGUMES	FIBER IN GRAMS
Baked Beans (1 C)	7.2
Black Beans (1 C cooked)	7.0
Chickpeas (1 C cooked)	18.2
Kidney Beans (1 C cooked)	19.4
Lentils (1 C cooked)	14.8
Lima Beans (1 C cooked)	14.8
Pinto Beans (1 C cooked)	17.8
Split Peas (1 C cooked)	10.2
White Beans (1 C cooked)	15.8

GRAINS, CEREALS, BREADS AND PASTAS

Most everyone loves a good bread and a hearty cereal. Just by changing the type of bread we feed our families can dramatically improve our fiber intake. Children that are raised on good whole grain breads instinctively turn away from sticky white bread. Breads which contain whole grained flours (stone milled is even better) and cereals with bran have the highest fiber content.

FOOD   **FIBER IN GRAMS**

BREADS

Bagel (1 medium)	1.2
Biscuit (1 small)	trace
Breads* (1 slice)	
Cracked Wheat	1.0
French	.7
Pumpernickle	1.4
Raisin	.7
Rye	.7
Whole Wheat	1.5

*The fiber count for these breads is low. I purchase breads which are readily available in grocery store bakeries that have 3 to 5 grams of fiber per slice.

CEREALS (3/4 C cooked)

Cream of Rice	.1
Farina	.7
Oatmeal	2.9
Wheatena	4.5

CEREALS (ready to eat)

All-Bran (1/3 C)	8.6
Bran Buds (1/3 C)	7.8
Cheerios (1 oz.)	1.1
Grapenuts (1/4 C)	1.4
Raisin Bran (1/2 C)	4.0
Fruit Loops (1 oz)	.2
Nature Valley Granola (1/4 C)	1.0
Life (2/3 C)	.9
Shredded Wheat (1 biscuit)	4.0
Total (1 1/4 C)	2.0
Wheat Chex (1 1/4 C)	2.1
Wheaties (1 1/4 C)	2.0
Cornmeal, (1 C dry)	19.8
Flour (1 C sifted)	
All-purpose	3.2
Rye	2.9
Whole Wheat	13.0
Grits (1/2 C cooked)	1.1
Macaroni (1/2 C cooked)	1.1
Muffins (1 average 3")	
Blueberry	.3
Bran	3.9
Corn	1.2
English	.3
Noodles (1/2 C cooked)	.7
Rice	
(1/2 C brown)	
dry	7.0
cooked	2.2

(1/2 C white)
    dry   2.1
    cooked   .7

Rolls

    White (1 large)   .7
    Whole Wheat (1 medium) 1.6

Saltines (1)   trace
Spaghetti or Pasta (1 C cooked) 2.1
Waffle (1)   trace

Wheat Bran (1 C)   23.8
Wheat Germ (3.5 oz.)   9.5

SNACK FOODS AND SWEETS

This is where we can really make a lot of progress if we would stop eating empty-calorie and fiber-poor junk foods and munch on snacks that are more nutritious and fiber-rich. Doughnuts, candy, candy bars, ice cream, most cookies, chips etc. are full of fat and have no substance. They clog our colons and fatten our frames so lets nix them once and for all. When you have a "hankerin" for something to nibble on reach for low fat or air popped popcorn, whole grain pretzels, raw nuts like almonds and pecans, raw sunflower seeds, carrot sticks etc. Use whole grain or bran in cookie and cake batters and try making your own whole wheat snack crackers. It's fun and a lot less expensive.

SNACK FOOD	FIBER IN GRAMS
Brownie (1)	.3
Cookies (1 medium)	
Chocolate Chip	trace
Fig Bar	.5
Raisin	.1
Corn Chips (10)	.2
Nuts	
Almonds (15)	2.1
Brazil Nuts (1/2 C)	3.1
Cashews (1/2 C)	2.4
Peanuts (1/2 C)	2.6
Pecans (1/2 C)	2.2
Walnuts (1/2 C)	1.6
Popcorn (1 C)	2.5

Potato Chips (10)	.2
Pretzels (10)	.1
Pumpkin Seeds (1/4 C)	.7
Sunflower Seeds (1/4 C)	1.3

CHAPTER EIGHT:

DIETARY FIBER, DISEASE TREATMENT AND PREVENTION

Scientists are beginning to understand that the condition of the colon is intrinsically related to all body systems and can potentially affect numerous chronic diseases, including cancer. Zolton P. Rona, M.D., MSc. has stated:

> "...many degenerative diseases are brought about by toxins generated in the large bowel. Bacterial flora imbalance, putrefaction of undigested foods, parasitic and yeast infections may be at the bottom (excuse the pun) of many diseases."

What goes on way down there in your bowel may seem totally unrelated to the condition of your veins, your gallbladder, breasts or even your mental attitude. The truth is that how we expedite waste material from the body may be a predictor of our health. To a great extent, what we put in our mouths determines that predictor.

We've already discussed the types of diseases which seem to specifically target western cultures. High fat, high protein, low fiber diets exact a devastating toll on our health and will cause thousands of unnecessary deaths and an enormous amount of suffering.

Dr. Arbuthnot Lane, surgeon to the King of England, spent several years specializing in bowel problems. He noticed that after he removed diseased sections of the bowel, his patients experienced remarkable and unexpected cures of completely unrelated diseases, such as arthritis and goiter. These observations led to his belief that a causal relationship between a toxic colon and other organs of the body exists. His advice was to care for the bowel first through good, sound nutrition.

THE FIBER HYPOTHESIS:

Dr. Burkitt and Trowell formulated the following hypothesis which is simply that:

- a diet which is rich in foods which contain fiber or plant cell walls (legumes, whole grains, fruits and vegetables) can protect the human body against a wide variety of serious disease which have specifically attacked western cultures.

- a diet low in fiber or plant cell walls can cause the incidence of these western diseases.

FIBER CAN HELP PREVENT INTESTINAL TOXEMIA

The idea of intestinal toxemia is based on the belief that what you eat determines the kind of bacteria which will inhabit your bowel. For example; if you eat a lot of complex carbohydrates, which are usually fiber rich, and little protein, your intestinal flora will primarily consist of bacteria designed to metabolize carbohydrates.

On the other hand, if your diet is high in protein and low in complex carbohydrates, that bacteria will be of the proteolytic type which breaks down and decomposes protein. This type of bacteria (the bad guys) release harmful gases and toxins which can remain in the colon and find their way back onto the body. Unhealthy intestinal flora can create adverse chemical reactions which can result in the production of powerful toxins.

Eating refined foods, a lot of meat and little fiber causes delayed elimination. Consequently, poisons such as phenols form in the colon. Some health experts believe that the presence of phenol in the body can be linked to a whole host of diseases ranging from allergies to arthritis to cancer, back pain and even mental illness.

Boosting your fiber intake while reducing animal protein and fats can decrease the amount of proteolytic bacteria in the colon, which contributes to the putrefaction of food waste. Any food material which enters the colon is subject to breakdown by the bacterial flora of the colon. Dietary fiber, by definition, reaches the colon intact and is a major source of energy for the colonic bacteria." In addition, studies have shown that in as little as two weeks, intestinal microflora can be altered by increasing your intake of dietary fiber. Even when the bacteria stabilized, the fiber continued to enhance intestinal fermentation and reduce the pH content of the stool.[22]

Because dietary fiber affects several vital metabolic processes, eating enough of it is crucial to maintaining good health and preventing disease.

The following section will discuss diseases which are specifically impacted by the consumption of dietary fiber. They include:

Appendicitis
Breast Cancer
Colitis
Colon and Colo-rectal Cancer
Constipation

Coronary Heart Disease/Cholesterol
Crohn's Disease
Dental Carries
Diabetes
Diverticular Disease
Duodenal Ulcers
Gallstones
Hemorrhoids
Hiatal Hernia
Hypertension
Irritable Bowel Syndrome
Kidney Stones
Obesity
Periodontal Disease
Pernicious Anemia
Prostate Cancer
Rheumatoid Arthritis
Varicose Veins

These diseases are certainly serious enough, however, a lack of fiber has also been associated with other afflictions as well. They include: gout, autoimmune disorders, pernicious anemia, multiple sclerosis and various skin disorders.

APPENDICITIS

DEFINITION:

Appendicitis refers to an acute inflammation of the appendix which is the small finger-shaped tube which branches off the large intestine. It has no known function, however it does contain a large amount of lymph tissue which helps defend against local infection.

CAUSES:

While most doctors will agree that the cause of appendicitis is not always known, it sometimes results from an obstruction of the appendix (a clump of feces or pinworms). The closed end of the appendix becomes inflamed, swollen and infected. If gangrene sets in, the appendix may burst, a potentially fatal condition.

INCIDENCE:

Appendicitis affects approximately 200 per 100,000 people every year in the United States. It is not commonly seen in the very young or the very old.

FIBER CONNECTION:

While some scientists and health care practitioners have not wholeheartedly accepted the relationship between appendicitis and fiber consumption, the evidence is compelling. Appendectomies are the most common abdominal surgical emergency in the Western world and are comparatively rare in third-world countries. How much more obvious can it be? While attributing all appendicitis to low fiber diets may be too simplistic, the correlation is clear.

It's no coincidence that appendicitis was rare in Western populations until 1870 to 1880, when grains began to be commercially milled and refined and major dietary changes took place.[23]

A sluggish bowel which is the result of poor dietary fiber levels has been associated with appendicitis. Dr. Burkitt discovered that fiber is the only dietary factor which can significantly speed up the transit of feces through the bowel and lower pressure within the colon. Clinical evidence tells us that when pressure rises in the appendix, it becomes vulnerable to infection by bacteria. Fecoliths or hard lumps of fecal material that obstruct the appendix can certainly occur when the bowel is sluggish, when bowel movements are infrequent or incomplete or if stool consistency is unformed and dry.

A 1940 report stated that when healthy, young Americans added bran to their diets, the appendix, which was invisible before, became visible through barium x-rays.[24] Of further interest is the fact that when diets were forced to revert to the increased consumption of whole grains, such as was the case in World War II, the frequency of constipation and appendicitis decreased. You don't have to be a rocket scientist to realize that fiber expedites waste material through the colon, therefore, it must help prevent fecal obstruction of the appendix.

Interestingly, the notion that eating too much popcorn can cause appendicitis may be actually be true. Yes, popcorn is a fibrous food, but if it is randomly ingested as part of a generally low fiber diet, its coarse kernels might get hung up in the bowel, perhaps contributing to the formation of a fecalith. So, if you are a habitual popcorn eater make sure to drink plenty of water and consistently eat foods rich in fiber.

There is also some evidence that people who get appendicitis may be more prone to develop certain types of cancer including colon and breast. It is strongly speculated that diets high in fiber could significantly protect against both conditions. An investigation of Greek populations and the incidence of appendectomy was that "in patients with cancer of the breast and ovaries, the incidence of appendectomy was found to be very high."[25]

It may be true that most of us don't find the threat of appendicitis particularly menacing, but its link to fiber is very telling. It is one of many physiologic conditions which may be almost 100 percent preventable if diets were rich in fiber.

PREVENTION:

Get your fiber intake up to 35 grams a day, reduce your fat and animal protein and drink plenty of water. Making sure that you have a well functioning bowel is crucial to preventing the kind of scenario which causes appendicitis in the first place. Remember that bland diets high in sticky white flour, sugar and fats create the perfect mix of ingredients which can cause the formation of a fecalith. Keep that colon clean with "fibery" whole foods.

BREAST CANCER

DEFINITION:

Breast cancer refers to the presence of a malignant tumor in the breast tissue which usually causes the formation of a lump. The lump is frequently felt rather than seen. In 90 percent of breast cancer, only one breast is affected. This unchecked growth of tissue can spread to other body systems.

CAUSES:

Current theories concerning breast cancer have focused on hormonal influences and diet, which may be intrinsically related. Women who began their periods early, who had no children, who began menopause at a later age and who had mothers or sisters with breast cancer have an increased risk of breast cancer. The relationship of birth control pills, pollutants and high fat diets is also linked to the disease. Clearly, at this point, women are beginning to raise questions concerning breast cancer that go well beyond early detection and forms of treatment.

INCIDENCE:

Breast cancer is the most common cancer in women. One in every 14 women will develop breast cancer and one in 20 will die from it. Mortality from breast cancer has not experienced a significant change in this century, however, in the 1980's research suggested that deaths can be reduced by a third with regular mammographic examinations. Despite the value of regular screening, the statistics on breast cancer are alarming, to say the least.

YEAR	NEW CASES OF BREAST CANCER
1961	63,000
1968	65,000
1972	70,000
1974	89,000
1978	90,000
1980	108,000
1984	115,000
1986	123,000
1988	135,000
1989	142,000
1991	175,000
1992	180,000

FIBER CONNECTION:

Breast cancer is a relatively rare disease in Japan, where a low-fat diet which is heavy on cruciferous vegetables is the rule rather than the exception. What's fascinating is that Japanese women living in the United States who eat a typically American diet have the same rate of breast cancer as anyone else.[27]

While we might connect the value of a high fiber diet with cancer of the colon, however, most of us are unaware of its profound role in breast cancer prevention. Several studies have looked into the role of fiber-rich foods in preventing the disease. Twelve case-control studies found a significant decrease in breast cancer risk in women who ate the highest amount of dietary fiber. These studies also found that women who ate the lowest quantity of cereals, beta-carotene, fruits, and vegetables had the greatest risk of developing breast cancer.[28] Keep in mind that the average American woman eats around ten grams of fiber each day.

THE ESTROGEN CAPER

How in the world can fiber help protect the breasts from developing malignant tumors? Fiber contributes to this function in three very important ways each profoundly related to the action of estrogen:

1. Fiber can modify the action of circulating hormones such as estrogen which is intimately connected to breast cancer. In other words, eating fiber helps to rid the body of excess estrogen or "bad" estrogen which can initiate the formation of breast tumors. Eating plenty of vegetable fiber, grain fiber, and fiber from fruits and berries have been associated with low levels of several hormones including: testosterone, estrone, androstenedione and free estradiol.[29] We all know that we need hormones to sustain life, however, high levels of certain hormones which continually circulate in our blood streams have been linked to a number of serious diseases including breast and prostate cancer. Fiber helps control hormones that have gone awry.

2. Many fruits and vegetables contain phytochemicals which can actually inhibit the action of estradiol in women. Cruciferous plants which include broccoli and cabbage contain substances called indoles that can also keep bad estrogen in check. In addition, dietary fiber may also interfere with the development of breast tumors by creating mammary lignins, which are created when plant lignins are chemically changed in the colon by friendly bacteria.[30] Isn't it amazing how all of our body systems interrelate to help protect us from disease? Unfortunately, as we've continually stressed, if our colons are compromised, the complete system of defense can break down.

3. Fiber helps decrease transit time, and makes the stool heavier, thereby expediting the removal of cancer-causing substances, including estrogen from the body. Many women are unaware that a significant amount of estrogen is excreted in their bowel movements. These estrogens, which find their way into the intestines from the liver as a constituent of bile must be eliminated. Because this waste can sit in the bowel for 24 hours or more, estrogen can be reabsorbed back onto the body.[31] Fiber can help to prevent this phenomenon. Breast cells need estrogen to grow, so if we decrease the amount of circulating estrogen, we decrease our risk of breast cancer.

How many of us know that bad estrogen may be circulating and re-circulating in our bodies and that by eating fiber we can help rid ourselves of excess hormone? Studies have found a very important relationship between the fiber content of stool and lower estrogen levels in the body.[32]

WHAT KIND OF FIBER IS BEST TO REDUCE ESTROGEN LEVELS?

Several studies have concluded that just increasing your fiber intake may not be as important as what kind of fiber you choose to eat. Scientists have discovered that estrogen levels went down only when sufficient amounts of wheat bran was added to the diet. Because wheat bran is primarily an insoluble fiber this makes good sense. Insoluble fibers can bind much more readily to substances like estrogen.

RULE OF THUMB: Eat enough fiber that you can actually notice that your stool floats and has a transit time of less than two days. Use the charcoal or beet test to determine your transit time.

PREVENTION:

- Eat a low fat, high fiber diet that is rich in complex carbohydrates. Foods such as cabbage, broccoli, brussels sprouts, and cauliflower contain phytochemicals which inhibit potentially dangerous estrogens.
- Eat foods rich in fiber and potassium such as beans, sprouts, whole grains, almonds, sunflower seeds, lentils, split peas, parsley, blueberries, endive, oats, potatoes with skin, carrots and peaches.
- Eat insoluble fiber on a daily basis, ie; wheat bran.
- Use herbs which help to balance hormones such as Saw Palmetto and Dong Quai

COLITIS/IRRITABLE BOWEL SYNDROME

DEFINITION:

Another of several disorders linked to Western diets and lifestyles, colitis refers to an inflammation of the colon which bring on episodes of diarrhea or constipation. Anyone who has experienced the perils of colitis doesn't want to be located to far from a bathroom facility. Irritable Bowel Syndrome refers to a similar condition which does not have its origins in inflammation but in an overly sensitive colon which responds to stress.

CAUSES:

Colitis can be caused by infection or the prolonged use of antibiotics, however poor eating habits play an enormous role. If you have a faulty diet, eat rapidly, drink too much liquid with your meals and have a tendency to be high strung, you're a candidate for colitis. Food allergies may also be a factor.

INCIDENCE.

This ailment is twice as common in women as it is in men and usually starts in early adulthood. It is the most common disorder of the intestine and accounts for more than half the patients seen by gastroenterologists.

FIBER CONNECTION:

A few years ago, doctors prescribed bland diets for anyone suffering from colitis or irritable bowel syndrome. The notion that high fiber could help an irritated colon that vacillated from constipation to diarrhea didn't seem plausible. Today, medical doctors have finally realized that high fiber diets and bulk forming agents can effectively treat these types of colon disorders.[33] Using bran or substituting wholemeal bread for white bread resulted in a significant improvement in symptoms of people with irritable bowel syndrome.[34]

Gentle natural laxatives such as Citrucel are routinely prescribed by doctors for colitis. Some doctors have even used psyllium therapy although the citrus-based laxatives are considered somewhat more gentle. Clearly, while eating oat bran may not provide an overnight cure for an inflamed colon, it will eventually result in a much healthier one. The question as to why the colon became inflamed in the first place is rarely addressed by the medical establishment.

Again, while its beginning to sound like a broken record, a fiber-depleted diet is considered a major factor in developing colitis.[35] Anyone who gulps their food, has high stress levels and eats a low fiber diet is putting a great deal of pressure on their colon. Sufficient chewing activates enzymes in the saliva which help to digest food properly. The Captain Crunch, hamburger and french fry diet can lead to fiber depletion and colon irritation.

Pectin fibers are particularly good for an inflamed colon and should be eaten liberally. Dr. Danny Jacobs M.D. referring to colitis has said, "Apples are a marvelous source of pectin..."[36] Bulking up the stool is also great for both the constipation and diarrhea that accompany colitis and irritable bowel syndrome.

It's important to gradually switch to high fiber foods so that the colon can adjust. Be careful with popcorn...it can promote diarrhea and should not be eaten until the colon heals. Start with 1/2 cup of oat or wheat bran cereal and go from there. Work yourself up to 1 1/2 cups every day and add lots of raw fruits and steamed vegetables.

Slippery Elm, an herbal medicine is very good for soothing and healing the irritated mucous membranes of the bowel.

FIBER TIDBIT

A recent study demonstrated the effectiveness of psyllium and wheat bran on stool frequency and consistency in patients with irritable bowel syndrome.[37]

PREVENTION

- Eat a low-fat, high fiber diet. Emphasize: cabbage, carrots, yellow fruits, cantaloupe, fruits with pectin, such as apple and pears, kelp, agar, watermelon and cucumbers. Add bran or whole grains to your diet slowly and increase over a number of weeks. Keep your bowels functioning well. Drink plenty of water.
- Avoid colon irritants such as: heavy rich junk foods, salt, sugar and fried foods.
- Don't snarf your food or eat under stressful situations. Eat slowly and chew thoroughly
- Don't ever used laxatives derived from unnatural sources. Citrus pulp supplements and psyllium are recommended.
- Find out if you have a food intolerance to certain foods like dairy products and stay away from them.

CONSTIPATION

DEFINITION:

Here is a question of profound significance, "How often should a person have a bowel movement in order to maintain good health?" Hippocrates, the father of medicine believed that defecation should occur "twice or thrice" daily. Today, answers range from after every meal to four times per week.

Generally speaking, if you have less than four bowel movements per week and if those movements are unformed or difficult to pass, you can consider yourself constipated. Many natural health care advocates define constipation as anything less than one bowel movement per day. More women suffer from constipation than men.

Constipation is really more of a symptom that an actual disease. Technically speaking, constipation refers to a decrease in bowel movements or difficulty in passing the stool. American bowel patterns are not statistically impressive and testify to our deplorable lack of dietary fiber. In some cases, diarrhea can be considered a form of constipation. Constipation can lead to diverticular disease and hemorrhoids, not to mention a wide variety of ailments linked to long transit times and poorly formed stool.

WHAT GOES IN DOESN'T ALWAYS ALL COME OUT

Recently, the notion that you can have regular bowel movements and still be constipated has received more attention. This idea is based on the incomplete evacuation of the bowel even when bowel movements are frequent. This implies that waste residue builds up on the colon walls and is not properly excreted with the contraction of bowel muscle. In other words, it sticks and can lead to the development of bowel disorders and other diseases.

CAUSES:

While constipation can be caused by a lack of activity, certain drugs, and various diseases, the greatest cause by far is a dietary one. It's a well-established fact that typical American eating habits promote constipation. Americans buy more laxatives than any other nation on earth. That in itself should tell us something. You can be sure that the topic of bowel movements is rarely discussed in cultures where it is taken for granted. Here, it is a source of major concern and much fretting.

Sadly, most people will continue to spend, strain and suffer with constipation when all along, it could have been cured with a simple change in eating habits.

INCIDENCE:

Great segments of our population are severely addicted to laxatives because constipation has become a way of life here in America. Western diet and lifestyles have resulted in the acceptance of constipation as a "normal" part of living. The vast amount of over-the-counter laxatives we consume as a nation have a whole host of undesirable side effects including dependence and vitamin depletion. In the U.S. alone, annual sales of laxatives and stool softeners amount to $500 million per year.[38] If we are eating properly, our bodies should not need artificial stimuli in order to eliminate properly.

FIBER CONNECTION:

Adding fiber to your diet, especially wheat bran can help prevent and get rid of chronic constipation. Several studies have proven its effectiveness. The amount of fiber recommended for anyone who suffers from constipation is 40 grams per day. Remember that all wheat brans are not equally effective. Coarse bran is better. Cereal sources of fiber are better for constipation that fruit and vegetables, however a combination of these foods is ideal.

Eating foods like wheat or oat bran must become part of a daily routine in order to treat and prevent constipation. Adding a psyllium supplement can move things along if your diet is lacking. Learn to routinely eat figs, prunes, watermelon, carrots, sesame and sunflower seeds, and berries. Most importantly, eat whole grains and don't forget the bran.

NOTE: If you have added fiber to your diet and your constipation persists, you may have a muscular problem in bowel. See your physician.

PREVENTION:

- Start off by eating a cup of bran cereal and increase that amount to one and a half cups over the next several weeks. If you use bran alone, a quarter cup per day is recommended.
- Make sure to drink plenty of pure water, at least 6 to 8 glasses a day.
- Eat plenty of raw fruits and vegetables with their peelings. Okra is particularly helpful.
- If you need to use a fiber supplement, purchase a psyllium or citric pulp product. Make sure your fiber supplement is vegetable based. Don't use laxatives unless they are non-addicting such as Cascara Sagrada (an herbal laxative).
- Exercise regularly, at least three times a week for 20 minutes.
- Avoid dairy products, refined white flours, sugars and fatty meats.
- Replenish your supply of healthy bacteria with good sources of acidophilus (active culture yogurts, kefir, buttermilk or acidophilus supplements).

COLON AND COLO-RECTAL CANCER

DEFINITION:

Colon or colo-rectal cancer refers to malignant tumors or lymphomas of the large intestine or rectum.

CAUSES:

Because these types of cancer are considered Western diseases, the role of diet is extremely important. A high meat, high fat and low fiber diet encourages the production and concentration of carcinogenic substances in the bowel and rectum. A genetic predisposition to the disease also plays a role.

INCIDENCE:

Approximately half a million new cases of colon cancer are diagnosed every year world wide. In 1987, 60,00 Americans died from cancers of the colon, rectum and anus and around 145,000 new cases were reported.[39] In 1994, 70,000 men and 67,500 women were diagnosed with colon and rectum cancer. The National Cancer Institute predicted that 6 percent of 250 million U.S. citizens would eventually develop colon cancer and six million of them would die from it.[40]

THE FIBER CONNECTION:

There is perhaps, no disease which could benefit more from fiber than colon and colo-rectal cancer. Accordingly, there has never been a more serious reason to eat diets that are high in fiber and low in fat than the threat of this devastating disease.

The health of the colon or large intestine and the rectum is profoundly related to what we put in our mouths. If we're are genetically prone to the disease, then our dietary habits become even more crucial. The colon is nothing more than our large intestine and is about 5 to 7 feet long. After many scientific studies on the causal factors for colon cancer, the number one culprit is diet. Consider this statement:

"The vast majority of human colon cancers are due primarily to the chemicals that are byproducts of the decomposition of bacteria and excess dietary fat and bile in the colon. A low fiber diet contributes to colon cancer by slowing down the system so that these decomposition products linger in the colon for extended periods. This increases the length of time that these decomposed products are in contact with the colon and increases the amount that is absorbed into colon cells."[41]

Where have we heard that before? This notion that eating fiber helps to promote the cultivation of good bacteria and the ingibition of God is vital to understanding how to maintain our health. The state of our health is determined to a great degree by the kind of bacteria which inhabit our colons. Eating fatty meats, refined sugar and low fiber generates putrefactive bacteria which produce harmful, carcinogenic compounds.

If you eat a high fiber diet you make friendly bacteria like:

Lactobacillus acidophilus
Lactobacillus bulgarius
Lactobacillus bifidum

Bifidobacterium bifidus
Bifidobacterium longum

If you eat low fiber diets you make unfriendly bacteria like:

bifidobacteria
bactericides

What is really interesting is that when we balance out our diets with certain foods, even if we eat fats, we are afforded a certain amount of protection from developing colon as well as other cancers. Cultures like the Finns who eat a high fat diet but combine it with lots of fiber and active culture yogurts have a low incidence of colon cancer.[42]

Both Dr. Burkitt and Dr. Trowell discovered that the type of food eaten by Africans made its journey from the mouth to the colon in one day or less. It takes most of us a minimum of three days for the same trip and some systems suffering from a very serious lack of fiber take up to two weeks. Can you imagine the kinds of poisons created by waste material that has putrefied for that long?

The double whammy of a low fiber diet as it relates to colon cancer can be summed up by these two actions.

1. Low fiber eating means producing bad bacteria, which generate carcinogenic compounds in the colon.

2. Low fiber eating means harboring those compounds for long periods of time before they are expelled from the body.

Eating plenty of wheat bran or other types of cellulose can reduce our risk of colon cancer. It's that simple. Emphasize whole grains like wheat and barley and eat plenty of legumes like dried beans, split peas, and lentils. Oat bran, guar gum and raw fruits and vegetables are also excellent.

In relation to all cancers, the dietary goals for the United States by the year 2000 are:

- To reduce the incidence of obesity by 20 to 26 percent
- To reduce dietary fat intake to 30 percent
- To increase fruits and vegetable intake from two and half servings per day to five.[43]

FIBER TIDBIT

One clinical study interviewed over 600 people with colo-rectal cancer compared with 3000 members of a control group and found that colo-rectal cancer patients consumed less fruit, vegetables and cereals than the controls.[44]

PREVENTION

- Eat a high fiber diet which concentrates on whole grains, legumes, and raw fruits and vegetables. Cruciferous vegetables are particularly protective against cancer causing chemicals whether they originate from our diets or not. These include: cabbage, broccoli, kale, collards, turnip greens and brussels sprouts. Taking supplements which contain indoles is also highly recommended if you cannot seem to eat enough cruciferous vegetables.
- Take antioxidant supplements such as selenium, vitamin C, bioflavonoids, pycnogenol, vitamin E and beta-carotene.

- Use garlic or take garlic supplements.

- Fish oils and zinc have also been recommended for maintaining colon health.
- Make sure you get enough calcium which helps to neutralize the toxic effect of dietary fats.
- Take a good acidophilus supplement.
- Use a psyllium or citrus pulp supplement if constipation is a problem.
- Be aware of your bowel habits and don't let yourself become constipated.

CORONARY HEART DISEASE/ CHOLESTEROL

DEFINITION:

Coronary heart disease refers to damage which occurs in the heart when the coronary arteries become blocked or narrowed due to a build up of plaque or oxidized cholesterol.

CAUSES:

Cholesterol does not have to necessarily be a bad thing. As a buzz word of the last two decades, all of us have become "cholesterol aware" however, that awareness has not motivated the kind of dietary changes that could literally save our lives. Coronary heart disease results from too much oxidized cholesterol, which nestles into the linings of our arteries, reducing blood flow to the heart or even worse, breaking off and lodging in the heart or the brain causing heart attack or stroke. The major causes of coronary heart disease include:

Obesity
Smoking
High Protein, High Saturated Fat Diets
Lack of Exercise
High Blood Pressure
High Cholesterol Levels

INCIDENCE:

CHD is an extremely common disorder of developed nations and causes more deaths in the United States than any other disease. Sadly, this disease strikes down men and women who are in the prime of their lives and seem to otherwise be in good health. Like high blood pressure, which is a related disorder, it can be a silent killer. While it's true that mortality rates from CHD have declined over the last 20 years, the primary reason is due to better medical technology. CHD claims more than one million deaths every year. The number of Americans walking around with heart and artery disease is estimated at around 50 million. Many of these people are completely unaware of their conditions.

FIBER CONNECTION:

Coronary heart disease, which devastates our society was found to be literally absent in the rural communities of South Africa. One of the most significant factors in determining whether we will get heart disease or not is cholesterol. So many of us have become cholesterol phobics and have replaced butter with polyunsaturated margarine, stopped eating eggs, use corn oil etc. when we were told that certain fats were the culprit.

Now, as is frequently the case, new data is telling us that high levels of cholesterol are not solely the result of eating foods like butter and eggs...there's more to the story. Eating whole foods as nature designed them should not hurt our bodies, however, the enormous consumption of processed fats, refined foods and lack of fiber has upset our physiological apple cart which cannot deal with this glut of non-nutritive or fragmented twentieth-century foods.

Additionally, if all we do is to concentrate on removing the fats from our diet, we are creating an unbalanced diet which is not a healthy one. My Italian grandmother used olive oil liberally, she would use only butter and no margarine but she also ate plenty of legumes and greens (at almost every meal) and lived to a ripe old age.

REMEMBER: Perhaps it's not so important to totally eliminate certain foods as it is to balance them or use them in moderation.

FIBER TIDBIT

Ancel Keys observed that there was a much higher content of plasma cholesterol levels of men in Minnesota as compared to Naples, Italy which could not be explained by patterns of fatty acid or cholesterol intake. His study indicated that the Italians ate diets high in cereals, vegetables, legumes and fruits which seemed to control cholesterol levels even if they ate butter, meat etc.[45]

Foods that are rich in fiber such as oats and beans, gums, pectins and psyllium all significantly lower blood fats or cholesterol levels. Interestingly, wheat bran and cellulose or insoluble fibers were not as good as oat bran and bean foods. However, insoluble fibers, which hold a lot of water can decrease the transit time of the stool, which means that cholesterol absorption into the bloodstream would be less.[46]

In addition, when you eat a lot of fiber, you get rid of more bile. When less bile is returned to the liver, it kicks in and makes more bile acids which uses up cholesterol floating around in your blood, lowering your cholesterol level.[47]

Nearly a dozen studies conducted over the past decade have proven that oat bran lowers cholesterol levels. Soluble-fiber cereals are highly recommended as bad cholesterol busters. In addition, psyllium has also proven itself to be a cholesterol inhibitor.[48]

FIBER TIDBIT

The Journal of the American Medical Association stated in 1988.

"A broad public health approach to lowered cholesterol levels by additional dietary modifications, such as with soluble fiber, may be preferred to a medically oriented campaign that focuses on drug therapy."[49]

BRAVO! When the medical profession actually recommends a nutritive therapy over a drug one, we know that therapy must be incredibly impressive. By now, we've accrued a mountain of evidence that dietary fiber can lower blood lipids and decrease our risk of heart attack or stroke. In fact, fewer than five percent of men in the highest third for cereal fiber intake developed coronary heart disease.[50]

FIBER FACTS TO REMEMBER CONCERNING HEART DISEASE

1. Sources of soluble fiber can significantly reduce your risk of heart disease. These include: dried beans of all kinds, lentils, split peas, oat bran, rice bran, barley, psyllium, gums and pectins (wheat fiber, cellulose and lignin are not as good, however they speed transit time which can also remove excess cholesterol and lipids from the body).

2. Soy fiber has also shown promise in preventing arterial disease.

3. Fiber reduces cholesterol levels in a number of fascinating ways:

a. It delays the emptying our of stomach contents which results in less fat absorption.

b. It speeds transit time, which affects the breakdown and absorption of fats

c. It affects enzyme function from the pancreas, which results in separating enzymes from fats changing the way they breakdown.

d. Fiber alters the flow of lymph, which affects the rate in which fats enter into the circulation from the digestive system

e. Fiber influences the secretion if insulin which has a bearing on how lipids are broken down in the bloodstream and stored.[51]

PREVENTION:

- By incorporating 100 grams of either oat bran or dried beans into your diet a significant reduction in LDL cholesterol levels can occur.
- Take a good fiber supplement to help control cholesterol levels, keep the colon clear and manage the appetite.
- Don't ever start smoking and if you do, quit.
- Exercise at least 3 times a week for 20 minutes.
- Don't become overweight.
- Avoid: processed foods, salt, white sugar, white flour, high protein fatty foods, and saturated fats (eating foods in moderation, in their natural state may be the key to balancing out all nutrients so none of them behaves bizarrely in the body).

DIABETES

DEFINITION:

Type one diabetes results when insufficient levels of insulin produced by the pancreas cause blood sugar levels to stay elevated. Insulin opens the cell doors so than sugar can enter. Without it, the sugar stays circulating in the blood and can cause all kinds of cellular damage. Type two diabetes is strongly related to obesity. In this case, the pancreas produces insulin, however a lack of chemical receptors on the cells makes them them insulin resistent so the sugar doesn't enter.

CAUSES:

Heredity plays an important role in both types of diabetes. Type one diabetes is commonly triggered after a viral infection or traumatic injury. Type two diabetes is closely related to obesity.

Some clinicians believe that fiber-depleted diets that are typically high in refined, processed foods have greatly contributed to the development of diabetes in our society.

INCIDENCE

Approximately two people for every 1000 have type one diabetes by the time they are 20 years old. Type two diabetes affects an estimated 5.5 million Americans. Around 2000 people for every 100,000 are affected.

FIBER CONNECTION

In 1679, Thomas Willis wrote, "Diabetes was so rare among the ancients that many famous physicians made no mention of it and Galen knew of only two sick of it."[52] From the years of 1866 to 1923, an early study noted that while the overall death rate declined a steady and impressive rise in diabetes death rates occurred.[53]

The idea that refined sugar and simple carbohydrates have played a role in the development of diabetes is based on observing a correlation between sugar consumption in various countries and the incidence of the disease. What has emerged is that while consuming sugar is certainly an important factor, the amount of fiber consumed along with that sugar may even be more vital.[54] If carbohydrates like maize or millet are eaten in their whole form, which is high in dietary fiber, blood sugar levels rise much slower. Interestingly, diabetes emerged as a common disease in India after the emergence of white rice, which is very low in dietary fiber.

In 1942, when cereal shortages necessitated the introduction of high fiber flour to replace white flour, diabetes mortality rates began to fall and continued to do so until 1954.[55]

By the mid 1970's, a number of clinical sutides had already concluded that increasing the amount of fiber consumed has a desireable effect on diabetics. Despite this evidence, doctors routinely prescribe low carbohydrate diets but rarely emphasize the blood sugar lowering effects of fiber.

FIBER HELPS THE BODY COPE WITH LARGE AMOUNTS OF SUGAR

Fiber slows the absorption of food in the small intestine. The rate in which carbohydrates are digested is closely related to how fast they are absorbed, which determines the rise of blood sugar. When carbohydrate and plant fibers are eaten together, blood sugar levels are considerably lower that when the same type of carbohydrate is eaten alone.[56]

This explains why so many of the sugary, highly refined cold cereals we feed our children can cause dramatic surges in blood sugar. Have you ever looked closed at a sugar smack or a fruit loop? The cereal mix has been so finely pulverized and refined it's hardly recognizable as a food. To make matters worse, adding enormous amount of white sugar to this mutated carbohydrate makes it behave like an injection of glucose when its consumed. Can you imagine how quickly a serving of chewed Captain Crunch is evacuated out of the stomach and how quickly it is absorbed. Virtually fiberless, it contains no balancing ingredients that would slow this process.

The fact that so many people suffer from what is referred to as hypoglycemia testifies to the fact that we are bombarding our bodies with simple sugars without the benefits of fiber. Hypoglycemia indicates the presence of an overly stimulated pancreas, which can eventually lead to its demise.

The average American consumes over 125 pounds of white sugar every year. Sugar makes up 24 percent of our daily calorie intake, with soda pop supplying the majority of sugar. As a nation, we eat an average of 15 quarts of ice cream per person per year. Our diets are loaded with sugar, hidden or added from our first bowl of sugary cold cereal to our daily big gulps, pastries, chips and candy bars.

Our homes and work places are teeming with sugar and lacking in fiber. The human body was not set up to process such enormous quantities of sugar. What is really disturbing is that combining this high sugar diet with a lack of fiber makes it so much more harmful to us.

To compound the problem, we have fragmented foods, fruits, grains etc. which further hampers our ability to metabolize glucose. Laboratory studies have confirmed the bad news: removing fiber from food or physically disrupting it disturbs glucose level stability and enhances insulin response which results is rebound hypoglycemia.[57] In other words, if you drink large quantities of apple cider instead of eating a whole apple, your blood sugar can shoot sky high, creating a surge of insulin which brings it down to a quick low, making you desperately crave more sugar so the vicious cycle propagates itself.

In East Pakistan, where wheat wholemeal, leguminous seeds and vegetables make up the majority of caloric intake, one of the lowest prevalence of diabetes was observed.[58]

Guar gum has also proven itself as a blood sugar lowering fiber. Even when insulin doses were not altered, adding guar gum to the diet reduced the amount of sugar excreted in the urine.[59]

FIBER TIDBIT

Diabetes was a rare disease in the ancient empires of Rome and Greece where high fiber diets were the rule. It became common at the same time that obesity did in the British upper class of the eighteenth century.[60]

OBESITY, DIABETES AND FIBER

It's common knowledge that if you become overweight, your chances of becoming diabetic are significantly increased. Diabetes is a leading cause of death in overweight men and women. Anyone who is 6 to 20 percent above their ideal weight has a 6 to 12 times greater chance of becoming diabetic.

The role of fiber as it relates to obesity is discussed in detail in a later section.

WHAT CAN FIBER DO FOR DIABETES:

- It can reduce the amount of insulin needed by keeping blood sugar levels lower.

- It can lower cholesterol and lipid levels in the blood, which can become elevated in the presence of too much insulin.

- It can help to promote weight loss, which can even cure some cases of adult onset diabetes.

If you are suffering from adult onset diabetes, you may be interested to know that high fiber diets have lead to a discontinuance of insulin therapy in 60 percent of noninsulin-dependent diabetics.[61]

PREVENTION

- Don't become overweight. Eat a diet that is high in complex carbohydrates, fiber and raw fruits and vegetables.

- Take a fiber supplement to help create a feeling of fullness and to slow the rise of blood sugar.

- Stay away from refined white sugar, white flour and avoid alcohol.

- Make sure you get enough chromium is your diet.

- Exercise regularly. Harvard University researchers have found that vigorous exercise can significantly reduce the risk of adult-onset diabetes by one-third.

DIVERTICULAR DISEASE

DEFINITION:

Diverticular disease results when the mucous membranes of the colon become inflamed which causes them to form small pouches called diverticula in the large intestine.

CAUSES:

Chronic constipation can cause diverticulitis by increasing the pressure in the bowel, which can cause blown-out pouch-like areas to form. The presence of hard, dry stool aggravates this problem. The diverticula or pouches in and of themselves cause no noticeable symptoms, however they can trap waste matter and subsequently become infected causing cramping, tenderness on the left side that is relieved by passing gas or having a bowel movement, diarrhea, constipation and nausea. A diet that is fiber-poor, obesity, gallbladder disease and family predispositions can all increase the risk of developing diverticular disease. Irritable bowel syndrome can co-exist with diverticular disorders and causes many of the same symptoms.

INCIDENCE:

Diverticular disease, like so many of the other diseases we've discussed, is rare in developing countries. In Western Europe and the United States, it affects more than half the population by the time they reach the age of 80. The incidence of diverticular disease increases progressively with age.

Diverticular disease did not appear as a medical problem until the turn of the century, when refined foods and simple carbohydrates began to replace fiber-rich foods. Lack of dietary fiber or roughage plays an extremely important role in the development of this disease. Diverticular disease has been linked to varicose veins, hemorrhoids and hiatus hernia, all disorders which have a connection to fiber deficiencies.

Vegetarians who eat fiber rich diets had a much lower incidence of diverticular disease, however those vegetarians that just abstained from eating meat and subsisted on white flour products did not.[62]

PREVALENCE OF DIVERTICULAR DISEASE IN VEGETARIANS AND NON-VEGETARIANS

Percent with diverticular disease		Fiber consumption/grams
vegetarians	6%	41
non-vegetarians	25%	21

FIBER CONNECTION:

It's not coincidence that diverticular disease is extremely uncommon in African blacks. Dr. Burkitt discovered that Africans who came down with this disorder had moved to the cities and were eating highly refined foods. The rural areas of Eastern Europe, India and the Middle East rarely see diverticular disorders. The creation of this disease is one of the many aliments which resulted from the switch to fiber depleted foods. In 1917, Sir John Bland-Sutton remarked, "In the last ten years, acute diverticulitis is recognized with the same certainty as appendicitis and is a newly discovered bane of elders."[63] Keep in mind that diverticular disease only affects citizens of economically developed western nation (some progress). It is virtually unknown to communities who have not adopted western eating habits.

We know all too well by now that the amount of fiber in the diet directly affects intestinal transit time and the weight and consistency of the stool. Fiber is closely involved in determining pressures in the colon, which are responsible for creating diverticular pouches in the first place.

Consuming adequate fiber in the form of fiber supplementation, whole cereals such as wholemeal bread, brown rice, vegetables and fruit help to prevent diverticular disease by:

- creating a large volume of feces with a wider diameter which does not allow for the formation of diverticular pouches.

- fiber shortens transit time, and adds to the moisture content of the stool, which makes for soft bowel movements that do not require straining. Passing difficult bowel movements creates undesirable pressure in the colon causing sections to balloon out into diverticula.[64]

Consider the following quote from Dr. Trowell:

"Rats fed a high-fiber diet by Carlson and Hoelzel did not develop diverticula, while those fed a low-fiber diet developed diverticula in the colon, Hodgen fed rabbits on white bread, dairy products and sugar. They gained weight while their health deteriorated and they became constipated. Their intracolonic pressure rose and their colons became narrower."[65]

The existence of diverticula in the large intestine is a sad commentary on the price we pay for our fiber "famine." Diverticular pouches form only after the colon has struggled for a number of years trying to excrete its sticky, dry contents a condition which results from eating low-fiber foods.

FIBER THERAPY FOR DIVERTICULAR DISEASE

Several studies have found that replacing fiber in the diet of people who suffer from diverticular disease can relieve nearly 90% of their symptoms.[66] The *British Journal of Clinical Practice* puts it succinctly: A high fiber diet is an effective treatment for diverticular disease.[67] Dr. James Scala writes:

> "In 1973, I published a paper entitled `Fiber, the Forgotten Nutrient.' Five years later I was a speaker at the annual meeting of food technologists; a man asked to shake my hand. I was surprised and asked why. He explained that he had read my paper while in the hospital awaiting surgery for diverticulosis. He showed it to his physician and asked if he could go home and try a high fiber diet. His surgeon said his knife was always ready and to give the diet a try. Six years later the man had avoided surgery by simply following a high fiber diet."[68]

Cereal fiber is the most effective kind when treating this disorder. Watch for whole grain and fiber content and don't be fooled by fibery sounding cereals that are really fiber whimpy. Anyone who has diverticular disease or a history of the ailment should:

- take a good cereal based fiber supplement daily

- eat bran-containing cereals and plenty of fruit

- avoid refined sugar, white flour and bread and eat whole grain whenever possible

- adding bran to batters, breads etc. is also recommended.

NOTE: Just adding non-cereal fiber to your diet will not relieve the symptoms of diverticular disease. It must be cereal fiber. In addition, taking a couple of teaspoons of bran in the morning and then consuming doughnuts, soda pop and pizza will not cure diverticular disorders. Ideally, you should be eating at least 35 grams of fiber per day.

For years, people who suffered from diverticular symptoms and other bowel disorders were told that roughage would irritate the colon further. This is clearly not the case with so many colonic disorders which desperately need the cleansing effect of fiber to finally heal. "Bran becomes softer when wet...it relieved abdominal symptoms such as aching, heaviness and distention that are associated with diverticular disease."[69]

PREVENTION:

- avoid white flour, white sugar, dairy products and processed foods.

- replace simple carbohydrates with high fiber cereals, bran supplements (oat bran), legumes, fruits and vegetables.

- drink plenty of water and exercise regularly.
- think "whole grains" and make sure your bowel movements are regular.

- avoid constipation like the plague by eating nutritiously and using a cereal (gum or pectin) based supplement if necessary.

- if you are a vegetarian, make sure you eat plenty of legumes and whole grain foods.

GALLSTONES

DEFINITION:

Gallstones form when cholesterol crystallizes with bile in the gallbladder. Between one and ten stones may collect in this small sac. Symptoms may not occur until one of the stones becomes stuck in the bile duct.

CAUSES:

The alarmingly high incidence of gallstones in the United States is directly related to western dietary habits (where have we heard that before?) A high fat, high protein, refined carbohydrate diet which elevates blood cholesterol levels increases the risk of developing gallstones.

INCIDENCE:

The fact that gallbladder removal surgery is one of the most common operations in the United States gives us some idea of how prevalent gallstones are. Over 20 million people suffer from gallstones, with at least 1 million new cases diagnosed each year.

Gallstones, along with just about every other disease discussed in this book, are rarely found in primitive cultures and again painfully point to the perils of western life styles and diet. Chronic constipation and obesity are considered risk factors for gallstones.

FIBER CONNECTION:

In the seventies, a hypothesis was presented that eating refined, fiber poor foods suppressed the liver's ability to make bile acids which resulted in less bile. The less bile, the more the contents of the gallbladder stagnate...the more stagnation, the higher the risk of stone formation. The addition of cholesterol rich foods only compounded the problem elevating lipids in the gallbladder which became bound to the bile acids and formed more stones. Now, to really make matters worse, if waste material stayed in the colon too long, toxic bile acid metabolites were re-absorbed into the body, causing the production of bile to be further impaired.[70]

The story doesn't end there...if you eat a fiber depleted refined carbohydrate diet, you have a tendency to become obese, which increases cholesterol synthesis and secretion even more.

Here's the clincher...the incidence of gallstones is related to: coronary heart disease, diabetes, obesity, diverticular disease, hiatal hernia and cancer. Every one of these diseases can be linked to low fiber, high fat diets. Could the message be any clearer?

Simply put: fiber depleted foods are a risk factor for gallstones. Technically, eating fiber helps to keep the bile acid pool from shrinking and at the same time helps to reduce blood serum cholesterol levels. By so doing, the two major components of gallstone formation are kept under control.

Scientific studies with animals have confirmed that the highest incidence of gallstones is found in animals who ate low fiber diets. Dietary fiber:

- reduces bile cholesterol concentrations
- keeps the bile acid pool active which discourages the formation of stones
- helps to prevent obesity which is significantly linked to gallbladder disease
- helps to bind with toxic bile acid metabolites in the colon keeping them from being reabsorbed into the bloodstream

Supplementing the diet with fiber such as wheat bran can actually help to leach out cholesterol from the liver as it crosses the portal blood to the bile.[71] Referring to our chapter on cholesterol and fiber further supports its crucial role in normalizing blood lipids.

THE CASE FOR EATING BREAKFAST

Something as simple as consistently missing breakfast is believed to increase the risk, of gallstones. Apparently, after fasting through the night, the gallbladder becomes more saturated with cholesterol because its bile content is retained too long, making the formation of crystals more likely. If constipation is considered one of the risk factors for gallstones then missing breakfast could also keeps the bowels quiet through the morning hours, retaining toxic bile metabolites in the colon. In addition, if we're going to eat fiber, we'll usually do it at the breakfast meal. Most of us rarely feast on oat bran for lunch or dinner.

NOTE: The types of fiber that have been tested for their effect on the gallbladder include wheat bran, lignin fibers and barley fiber.

PREVENTION:

NOTE: Gallstones are much easier to prevent than to treat.

- Emphasize the following foods: fiber (oat bran, flaxseed, guar gum, pectin, psyllium), vegetable proteins such as soy, legumes, fresh fruits and vegetables and plenty of water.

- Do not become constipated. Retaining stool in the bowel can increase your chances of gallbladder disease. Take a natural fiber supplement if necessary.

- Do not become overweight. Even slightly overweight people have twice the risk of developing gallstones. Lose weight safely and slowly, Losing weight too quickly with drastic diets can actually increase your risk of developing gallstones. An extremely low-fat diet or one that uses fasting can cause bile to sit in the gallbladder too long, making stone formation more likely.

- Avoid saturated fats and foods high in cholesterol. Use vegetable proteins instead of animal sources. Minimize your consumption of fatty, dairy foods also.

HEMORRHOIDS

DEFINITION:

A hemorrhoid is nothing more than a varicose vein located in the anal region. These distended veins can swell and protrude causing pain and itching.

CAUSES:

Repeatedly straining to move hard dry feces typically causes hemorrhoids although they can occur as a complication of pregnancy and childbirth. Our dependence on laxatives attests that millions of our citizens are constipated and rarely have healthy bowel movements Dr. Burkitt observed among rural Africans.

INCIDENCE:

It has been estimated that approximately one in two Americans over the age of 50 suffers at some time or another from hemorrhoids which has become almost as common as cavities. Hemorrhoids are relatively rare in third world countries (here we go again). You don't have to be a genius to realize that dietary habits predict, to a great degree, the prevalence of hemorrhoids.

FIBER CONNECTION:

A low fiber diet causes the stool to become unformed, hard and dry. Straining during a bowel movement causes venous pressure to rise making veins more vulnerable to injury when stressed. When you have to force a bowel movement, delicate mucous membranes can become damaged. These swollen veins can bleed, causing all kinds of discomfort.

A lack of fiber, especially cereal fiber can cause the formation of hard feces. Eating high fiber foods or using vegetable based fiber supplements result in a soft, formed stool which can pass easily without straining.

Even people who have been suffering from constipation for years will be surprised to find that a relatively simple change in their eating habits can produce a dramatic improvement in their bowel function.

"There is no doubt that increasing fiber intake to make defecation easy is often sufficient to stop bleeding, and reduce the incidence of prolapse. Since all patients with hemorrhoids have been encouraged to go on a high fiber diet for life, I have found that few of them have any further trouble after their initial treatment."[72]

Additional studies have confirmed that adding bran to the diet improves stool bulk, decreases transit time, encourages the healing of hemorrhoids and discourages their recurrence.[73] In addition, if you're treating your hemorrhoids with medications or recovering from a hemorrhoidectomy, you'll recover sooner if your boost your fiber intake.

It's hard to believe the amount of damage that western eating habits have inflicted on human physiology. Obviously, hemorrhoids, like so many of the other ailments we've talked about prove, once again, that our intestinal system depends on fiber to remain toned and functional.

PREVENTION:

- Eat plenty of high fiber foods including: oat bran, wheat bran, whole grains, raw fruits and vegetables, dried prunes, dates and legumes.

- Avoid the empty calories found in refined food diets. Simple carbohydrates do not adequately bulk up the stool and can cause straining during bowel movements.

- Guar gum and psyllium are natural bulking agents that can significantly reduce constipation and straining.

- Drink 6 to 8 glasses of water each day.

HIATAL HERNIA

DEFINITION:

Hiatal hernia refers to a condition in which a portion of the stomach protrudes upward into the chest through a hiatus (opening) in the diaphragm which separates the chest from the abdomen. Small hernias often go undetected. Persistent heartburn and belching are considered indicators of the disorder.

CAUSES:

Most medical texts will cite that the underlying cause of a hiatal hernia remains somewhat of a mystery. They do know that it tends to occur in obese people and in upper middle-aged women, and that it can result from pregnancy.

It is believed to be caused by an increase in intra-abdominal pressure. Its connection to pressure created by straining to move hard feces is rarely discussed. As is the case with hemorrhoids, consistently forcing the muscles to bear down in order to move the stool creates an enormous amount of pressure which wreaks all kind of havoc with living tissue. Some may claim that the link between habitual constipation and hiatal hernia has not been scientifically established. Look at the facts and draw your own conclusions.

NOTE: Our western style toilet seats may not be doing us any favors. People in developing countries who squat when they have a bowel movement are afforded more natural protection to the diaphragm than sitting on a raised toilet seat.[74]

INCIDENCE:

It has been estimated that fifty percent of the population over forty suffer from a hiatal hernia. In 1926, the incidence of hiatal hernia was reported as 2 to 3% of al upper gastrointestinal tract examinations. By 1950, the figure had risen to 15% and since then has substantially increased.[75] To give you an idea of how uncommon this disorder is in third world countries, it isn't even listed in some medical textbooks. During the sixties in Kenya, doctors detected only one case of hiatal hernia in 1314 barium x-ray examinations.[76]

FIBER CONNECTION:

Like hemorrhoids, hiatal hernia is believed to be linked to what we eat and how we get rid of waste material from the body. Medically speaking, the intra-abdominal pressure caused by bowel movement straining can actually exceed intra-thoracic pressure which can force the gastro-esophagal junction upward into the chest cavity. Is that technical enough for you? What this means in simple lay terms is, don't get constipated.

By now, we have firmly entrenched into our consciousness the fact that eating a low fiber diet can cause hard, dry feces. In relation to hiatal hernias, keep in mind the following facts:

1. Cultures that eat high fiber foods have a very low incidence of hiatal hernia.

2. People who eat fiber-rich foods have frequent bowel movements, shorter transit times and have soft, formed stool.

3. A lack of cereal fiber can significantly reduce the ability of the diet to form bulk.

4. Western eating habits including a high intake of dietary fat, smoking and alcohol all affect the lower esophageal sphincter which is involved in hiatal hernia.

Recent studies have concluded that a low-fiber diet can increase one's risk for hiatal hernia.[77]

PREVENTION:

• Keep your weight down. Becoming obese can increase pressure on the abdominal cavity.

• Prevent constipation by eating a fiber-rich diet and taking fiber supplements if necessary.

• Eat a diet low in fats, (fried foods, fatty dairy products, fatty meats) and watch out for overly large portions.

• Don't smoke or use alcohol. Both of these habits have been linked to lowering esophageal sphincter pressure which could lead to a hiatal hernia.

NOTE: Hiatal hernia, gallbladder disease and diverticular disease are referred to as the "saint's triad" and are intrinsically linked in their geographical distribution and their common denominators. If you get gallstones, you have a better chance of getting a hiatal hernia and vice versa.[78] All of the fascinating links that we've seen between so many of these diseases point to the low fiber factor, which is shared by them all.

HYPERTENSION

DEFINITION:

Having high blood pressure should never be taken lightly. Hypertension is considered one of the major medical problems of our age and like so many of the diseases we've talked about, it is considered a liability of 20th century lifestyles and diet. Of all the risk factors, high blood pressure is the most accurate predictor of future cardiovascular disease in people over the age of 65. Technically, hypertension refers to a condition where too much pressure is exerted against the arterial walls. If the arteries become constricted or blocked, then each time the heart forces blood into the system, pressure will mount. You can imagine the strain that the heart experiences as pressure increases and pumping becomes more difficult.

CAUSES:

High blood pressure runs in families and has been linked to smoking, obesity, hardening of the arteries and heart disease. If you have a tendency to retain water, your blood pressure will also become elevated. Kidney disease and hormonal disruptions can also cause hypertension. A whole host of over-the-counter and prescription drugs may also result in an elevation of blood pressure. Cardiovascular disease and obesity are by far the greatest factors associated with hypertension and have been directly linked to dietary habits. Some people have the kind of blood pressure that cannot be traced to any identifiable cause.

INCIDENCE:

The incidence of high blood pressure dramatically increases with age and is twice as high among Afro-Americans. Blood pressure medications are some of the most widely prescribed drugs in our country and come with a number of undesirable side effects.

FIBER CONNECTION:

The role of fiber as it affects hypertension has not been adequately addressed. Surprisingly, the role of dietary fiber as it relates to high blood pressure has received little attention. Eating a fiber-rich diet most definitely affects hypertension. The fact alone that vegetarians have lower blood pressure than control groups can clearly be interpreted as being a reflection of fiber intake to some degree.[79]

Recent double-blind placebo controlled clinical tests have confirmed that taking fiber supplements significantly reduces diastolic blood pressure in obese women.[80] In addition, taking fiber therapeutically also reduces blood pressure in normal as well as overweight people who suffer from hypertension.

Clearly, the profound role that fiber plays in controlling weight is also intrinsically linked to high blood pressure disease. Additionally, its profound role in keeping cholesterol levels down directly affects the health of arteries, which when they collect plaque, become narrow and increase blood pressure.

Some health practitioners strongly believe that a low-sodium, low fat, high fiber diet can be more useful in treating hypertension than any single dietary approach.[81] Various studies have discovered that just by increasing your high fiber cereal consumption, you can reduce your blood pressure. It's no accident that people who eat high fiber diets have lower blood pressures than those who don't. Like so many of the physiological functions that are affected by fiber, one system profoundly influences another. Hypertension is a great example of a condition that is related to weight, cholesterol and other factors that can be controlled by a fiber-rich diet.

PREVENTION:

- Emphasize a low fat, high fiber diet. Eat plenty of oat bran, pectin fruits, bananas, apples, melons, broccoli, cabbage, green leafy vegetables, peas, beets, carrots and essential fatty acids.

- Eat a low fat, low salt diet.

- Do not smoke. Smoking is directly linked with the development of coronary artery disease.

- Do not consume alcohol.

- Don't drink water that has been softened.

- Learn to manage stress with meditation, massage, music etc.

INFECTION

DEFINITION:

The term infection refers to the invasion of body cells by either viral or bacterial organisms which can multiply causing a whole host of symptoms including fever and inflammation. Infectious diseases are a large and important group of conditions, and until recently, were a major cause of illness and death throughout the world. While vaccines and antibiotics have greatly curbed certain infections, we are currently seeing the development of new viral and bacterial strains, some of which are antibiotic-resistant. It is for this reason that the notion of strengthening the immune system to resist and fight infection has become as vital as treating the infection after the fact.

CAUSES:

Disease causing organisms fall into a number of well-defined groups including viruses, bacteria, and fungi. All of these are relatively simple organisms and can readily multiply in human tissue.

INCIDENCE:

While the incidence of some infectious diseases such as poliomyelitis, smallpox, diphtheria and tuberculosis dramatically declined over the last century, these diseases are currently experiencing a resurgence to some degree. In addition, the prevalence of AIDS and other incurable and potentially fatal viruses have emerged over the last few decades. The Ebola virus and other related strains are extremely difficult to treat with antibiotics. Some health experts believe that we are only one antibiotic away from an infectious epidemic which will not respond to current medications. For this reason, boosting immunity is crucial. Those of us who have supported our immune system may actually be exposed to carcinogens and pathogens which do not result in disease. To the contrary, someone who has not nutritionally invested in their physical health may become infected through the same exposure.

FIBER CONNECTION:

Some studies have concluded that pectin and cellulose fibers may play a role in supporting the immune system. In addition, fiber helps to stabilize blood sugar levels. High blood sugar can leave one susceptible to all kind of infections especially fungal ones like yeast.

The intrinsic connection between eating fiber and maintaining good intestinal flora is also very important for our immune defenses. Eating fiber helps us to make the friendly bacteria which fight off antagonistic varieties. Eating low fiber, refined, processed high protein foods does just the opposite.

The presence of fiber in the gastrointestinal tract also helps to expedite substances such as mucus out of the body, which may actually trap infectious organisms like as parasites in the intestine. Interestingly, animal studies have found that even after an infection has been initiated, eating high fiber foods can decrease the length of that infection.[82]

So, eating creamed, white, floury soups, milk shakes and white bread are definitely not recommended as immune system booster foods. Think whole grains, raw fruits, vegetables and drink plenty of pure water.

PROSTATE CANCER

DEFINITION

Prostate cancer occurs when a malignant growth forms in the outer zone of the prostate gland. Unfortunately, the symptoms of prostate cancer can be rather vague. Consequently, approximately 90 percent of prostate cancer goes undetected until it has progressed to a much more serious stage which is difficult to treat.

CAUSES

Developing prostate cancer has been linked to several factors, however its dietary connection has recently been strengthened. What men choose to eat has a profound effect on their prostate health status. In addition, a history of venereal disease and chronic prostate infections also are associated with an increased risk of prostate cancer.

INCIDENCE

Statistics indicate that 103 men in a thousand will develop prostate cancer. In 1993, 132,000 men were diagnosed with prostate cancer and 34,000 of them died from it. The incidence of prostate cancer has escalated by 39 percent since 1973.

FIBER CONNECTION

The similarities between breast cancer in women and prostate cancer in men is currently being explored. Both of these cancers are related in that they can be hormonally induced. In addition, inhibiting certain "bad" forms of estrogen and testosterone can significantly reduce the risk of developing these cancers.

Eating a high fat diet in combination with refined white sugars and flours increases the risk of prostate disease including cancer. On the other hand, eating a diet that is high in natural whole grains, fresh fruits and vegetables and low in saturated fat can help support the prostate gland and encourage both healing and protection.

High fiber foods are particularly good for their ability to rid the body of bad hormones which encourage the formation of breast and prostate tumors. Like we mentioned before, these carcinogenic hormones can be retained in the bowel if transit time is too slow and re-circulate through the bloodstream, stimulating the growth of malignancies in the breast and prostate gland.

Foods like whole oats, brown rice, whole wheat, millet, barely and buckwheat are recommended. If you need to add bran or any good natural fiber supplement to your diet. Cultures who routinely eat high fiber foods have a low incidence of all kinds of cancer, including the prostate variety.

Flaxseeds are a good source of fiber and essential fatty acids which help to regulate and protect the prostate gland.

PREVENTION

- Maintain a whole food diet and supplement with zinc and flaxseed oil.

- Eat plenty of raw nuts and seeds (especially pumpkin seed, raw vegetables, fruits, dried beans, peas and brown rice.

- Avoid eating refined and processed foods, coffee, strong tea and alcohol, which have all been linked to cancer of the prostate.

ULCERS

DEFINITION

Technically, an ulcer is an open sore that forms on the mucous membrane lining of the stomach. It may be shallow or deep and is characterized by pain and inflammation. Most ulcers are found within the upper digestive tract and are comprised of peptic, duodenal and gastric ulcers.

CAUSES

Stomach ulcers occur when the mucous lining that normally protects the stomach from the damaging effects of stomach acid breaks down. While factors such as stress and eating certain foods have been related to the formation of ulcers, the exact reason why the mucous lining becomes weak in the first place has prompted new ulcer therapies. The current view is that ulcers are bacterially caused. Apparently, it is the invasion of certain bacteria which causes the mucosal lining to weaken. Smoking and taking certain drugs can also make you more prone to developing an ulcer.

Unquestionably, our eating habits, what and how we eat play a significant role in predisposing us or protecting us from ulcers.

Medical views on the proper treatment for ulcers have changed over the last few years. Doctors no longer advise their ulcer patients to drink whole milk or rich dairy products to neutralize excess stomach acid. The truth has recently surfaced that eating fatty dairy products will only cause the stomach to secrete more acid.

INCIDENCE

An estimated 5 million Americans suffer from ulcers. Even when ulcers heal, their chances of recurrence are high.

FIBER CONNECTION

Recent studies strongly suggest that a connection exists between eating low fiber diets and developing stomach ulcers. Statistics point to the fact that rice bran and unprocessed rice has the ability to protect the stomach lining from ulcer formation. The therapeutic use of guar gum to heal ulcerated stomach tissue has shown some impressive results. Guar gum also acts as an effective stomach protectant.[83]

If ulcers are bacterially caused, the ingestion of high fiber foods may also play a role in the way that food is digested, thus contributing to stomach resistance or susceptibility to microorganism invasion. We already know that fibery foods can expedite the removal of pathogens from the gastrointestinal tract and boost friendly bacteria proliferation. Both of these factors determine, to a great degree, whether we fight off or become vulnerable to any kind of infectious disease. In addition, fiber rich foods promote the secretion of mucin which acts as a protectant against ulcer formation. It is also good to know that barley helps rebuild the lining of the stomach.

NOTE: Several fruits and vegetables have been associated with a lower risk of stomach cancer. These include: fresh fruit, onions, tomatoes, celery and squash. Interestingly, canned, cooked fruits have been linked to an increased risk for stomach cancer.[84]

PREVENTION

- Avoid highly processed, refined, fatty foods and emphasize whole grains, raw nuts and seeds, fresh vegetables and fruits. Cabbage is thought to be especially healing to stomach tissue and contains nature's wonderful indoles, which are believed to protect cells from cancer.

- Don't smoke. Smoking constricts the blood vessels that supply nourishment to the stomach lining.

- Avoid alcohol which can irritate the stomach lining.

- Supplement your high fiber diet with zinc and garlic.

VARICOSE VEINS

DEFINITION

Varicose veins are vessels which have become swollen due to a weakness in the vein wall or valve, allowing for a backflow of blood to occur. As a result, blood pools in superficial veins, causing them to become stretched and puffy. The legs are more susceptible than any other area to varicose vein development. Spider veins, which are usually found in the thighs are a much milder form of varicose vein.

CAUSES

Varicose veins can be aggravated by a lack of good circulation which results in the twisting and dilating of veins. Pregnancy or prolonged standing have been associated with the development of varicose veins. It is important to understand that these components are secondary not primary causal factors. In other words, while certain situations make it easier to generate varicose veins, other, more important reasons determine their existence.

Hemorrhoids are nothing but anal varicose veins and also result from too much venous pressure. Straining to pass hard bowel movements can also contribute to the formation of varicose veins in the legs as well as the anus.

INCIDENCE

More than 40 million Americans suffer from varicose veins with women outnumbering men four to one. Varicose veins are one of the most common disorders that surgeons confront and their prevalence is rising.

Varicose veins are so common that they rarely receive the serious attention they merit. Ask anyone who suffers from unsightly, varicose veins just how troublesome the problem is to them.

FIBER CONNECTION

Varicose veins are seldom seen in areas of the world where high-fiber diets are the rule. Typical western dietary habits unquestionably contribute to the development of varicose veins.

Dr. Burkitt questioned doctors in over 200 hospitals in nearly 50 countries and found that the incidence of varicose veins was practically nil in Asia and Africa.[85] Again, the ultimate irony was that the more affluent the community, the greater the incidence of the disorder. The main factor that affected the prevalence of varicose veins in these communities was the degree of contact with Western civilizations.

Dr. Burkitt concluded that if pregnancy or standing too long caused varicose veins then the malady would be evenly distributed throughout the world. In fact, he postulated that there should be less varicose veins in Western cultures, where people could sit more throughout the course of a normal workday. Of the 1000 pregnant women he surveyed in India, only 1.1% of them experienced varicose veins.[86]

Burkitt discovered that communities with a very low incidence of varicose veins were the same ones who consistently had healthy and ample bowel movements. He concluded that when we get constipated, intra-abdominal pressure rises, which can cause abdominal straining. The one, most important cause of constipation so prevalent in the Western world was a lack of cereal fiber in the diet.

Isn't it interesting that people who eat the way nature

intended rarely suffer from varicose veins? Why don't animals get varicose veins? Again, we're back to the same old story....keep the bowels working smoothly and so many seemingly unrelated ailments will never have the chance to inflict their misery.

PREVENTION

- Emphasize a diet high in cereal fiber found in whole grains and add plenty of legumes, and fresh fruits and vegetables.

- Avoid fatty foods and refined carbohydrates. Stay away from margarine, red meat, and rich dairy products.

- Eat plenty of onion and garlic, and add vitamin C supplements to your diet.

- Exercise regularly.

CHAPTER NINE:

FIBER AND WEIGHT CONTROL

Running on Empty

The sad truth concerning weight control is that despite the glut of low-fat, non-fat, artificially sweetened, "lite" foods that crowd our grocery store shelves, AMERICANS ARE FATTER THAN EVER.

"...as of 1993, 68% of Americans were overweight, up from 58% a decade earlier..."[87]

"As many as 20% of children and 30% of adults in the United Sates are considered to be obese and the numbers appear to be increasing."[88]

Unfortunately, billions of dollars after the fact, weight reduction programs and artificially altered foods have not succeeded in maintaining ideal weights. To the contrary, drastic diets have initiated weight loss in the human body that has consistently resulted in compromising health and the pounds inevitably return.

"Two out of three people who go on a diet regain the weight in one year or less. 97% will regain the weight in five years."[89]

Simply stated, human physiology responds to dieting the same way it does to the potential threat of starvation...it turns the engines down. Consequently, it burns less fuel and stores it much more efficiently (thanks a lot). The very process of dieting can serve as a self-defeating exercise for those of us who battle the bulge. The concept of successful weight loss should go hand-in-hand with healthy, nutritious eating.

FIBER AND OBESITY

If we want to lose weight effectively and permanently we need to focus on the following goals:

- to cleanse the body of toxins which impair metabolic processes and are fostered by a sluggish colon

- to satisfy hunger and discourage food binging

- to regulate blood sugar levels so that hunger is normalized

- to provide energy and satiety so that we don't go rummaging through the pantry every two hours.

- to discourage the formation of future fat stores

- to provide nutritional support during thermogenesis

A diet that is high in fiber and emphasizes plenty of whole grains, raw fruits and vegetables and is low in protein and fats can help to meet the criteria listed above. Let's be painfully honest. Most of us have high accessibility to pastries, cookies, highly sugared soda pop, fast food places galore and we routinely eat inordinately large portions of food. The American concept of a good meal deal is "the bigger, the better."

We live in an incredibly prosperous society and rarely deny ourselves the vast array of fattening delectables that surround us on every side. We need to redirect our notions of what are appetizing or appealing foods and reach for unrefined, whole, nutritious foods.

FIBER TIDBIT

If we cannot consistently eat enough fiber through our selection of foods, we should consistently use a good, natural fiber supplement to keep weight in control.

SPECIFIC ACTIONS OF FIBER THAT PROMOTE WEIGHT LOSS

- increases saliva production
- increases chewing time
- increases gastric filling
- slows gastric emptying
- slows glucose absorption
- lowers insulin secretion
- increases fecal excretion

THE COLON'S CONNECTION TO WEIGHT LOSS

The status of our colon is rarely linked to obesity. The fact that weight reduction can be significantly inhibited by chronic constipation must be recognized. Here we go again: cultures that routinely eat high fiber diets have a very low incidence of obesity. Unquestionably, these people do not count calories to maintain their ideal weight.

Fiber reduces the absorption of fat by drawing water into the intestinal system which creates a sensation of fullness with less caloric intake. Studies have found that when high fiber diets are consumed over a period of time, food cravings will diminish.

NOTE: Many of our food cravings are not prompted by a true physiological nutrient need. When we eat refined and processed foods that shoot insulin into our blood streams, to compensate for high blood sugar, that level of blood sugar will inevitably take a dive. When that happens we'll do anything to satisfy our craving for a carbohydrate. Under these circumstances I've been known to rummage through the junk drawer for an old, stale chocolate.

DIETARY FIBER CAN PREVENT AND TREAT OBESITY BY:

1. Slowing down the eating process by increasing the amount of chewing required.

2. Increasing the excretion of fat in the feces.

3. Improving digestive hormone secretion which facilitates better digestion and reduces food intake.

4. Improving glucose tolerance which prevents wild blood sugar swings.

5. Creating a feeling of fullness or satiety.

FIBER SUPPLEMENTS AND WEIGHT LOSS

Using a good fiber supplement is highly recommended as a way to ensure that you're getting adequate amounts of soluble and insoluble dietary fiber. The best kinds of supplements utilize a combination of pectins, gums and brans.

In relation to weight loss, psyllium has an impressive track record. Because it is such a good bulking agent, psyllium supplements can significantly boost the process of weight loss.

"In Italy, a study on the effects of Plantain (psyllium) in a reducing diet for women who averaged about 60 percent overweight resulted in weight loss greater than that obtained by diet alone. The effects of psyllium on weight loss was dramatic. In summary, it appears that psyllium produces weight loss by limiting caloric intake, due to its appetite-satiating effect, and by reducing intestinal absorption of lipids."[90]

While psyllium-based supplements are good, guar and other gums are also excellent fiber sources and can effectively promote weight loss.

REMEMBER: TAKING A DAILY DOSE OF A FIBER SUPPLEMENT CAN EXPEDITE WEIGHT LOSS BY:

1. Increasing your feeling of fullness and discouraging food cravings and abnormal hunger surges.

2. Providing intestinal bulk which helps to clear lipids from the body without contributing one single calorie in the process.

*REMEMBER: FIBER SUPPLEMENTS CAN BE A DIETER'S BEST FRIEND.

TRY TO REDEFINE WHAT YOU WANT TO EAT AND WHY

The bottom line is that the types of foods we routinely eat are perfectly designed to put on weight. White flour, white sugar, fatty, processed foods are:

quickly digested
drastically raise blood sugar levels
create abnormal food cravings
encourage snacking
stick to the walls of the bowel
are high in calories and low in substance and
nutrition

Eat the whole apple rather than the apple juice, eat the potato peeling along with the potato, eat hardy, whole grain breads and start the day with a fiber rich cereal. Look over the recipes found in the back of this book to get menu ideas. High fiber eating can be absolutely delicious and very satisfying. It's the way we were meant to eat.

*REMEMBER: A FIBER RICH DIET FACILITATES WEIGHT LOSS IN A SLOW AND PERSISTENT WAY. FORGET QUICK WEIGHT LOSS SCHEMES AND RE-BALANCE YOUR METABOLISM THROUGH WHOLE, NATURAL FOODS THAT ARE LOW IN FAT.

CHAPTER TEN:

FIBER SUPPLEMENTS... ARE THEY NECESSARY?

Because most of us have good intentions but rarely meet our optimal dietary goals, fiber supplementation is recommended. Ideally, we should be eating enough "fibery" foods in the form of fruits, vegetables and whole grains. Realistically, we usually fall short, no matter how dedicated we might be. If we have any type of glucose impairment disorder like diabetes, we may not be able to eat the amount of fruit recommended.

We may never develop a taste for whole grain cereals (would be a real tragedy) or may be guilty of consistently meal skipping. If we are allergic to grains like wheat, obtaining enough fiber could be significantly more difficult.

For any or all of these reasons, finding a high quality fiber supplement is recommended. If you're going to purchase a fiber supplement, make sure that it's formula is vegetable based.

FIBER TIDBIT

If you insist on continuing with poor eating habits such as having a bowl of frosted flakes for breakfast, by adding a good fiber supplement to your "meal," you can beef up the whimpy flakes and give them some of the fiber punch they lack.

WATCHWORD: Taking a fiber supplement can never replace eating properly. Human physiology functions best when it is fueled with whole, unaltered foods that are naturally rich in fiber.

THE ADVANTAGES OF TAKING A FIBER SUPPLEMENT

1. It's an easy way to fortify your diet with fiber two to three times a day if desired.

2. Vegetable fibers that have been ground to powders can make the fiber source more digestible.

3. Fiber formulas can contain sources of fiber as well as other nutrients or herbs that we would not normally consume, ie: rice bran, guar gum, pectin, gum acacia, locust bean gum, psyllium, aloe vera, etc.

4. Fiber supplements sometimes contain a variety of fiber sources which are much more preferable than just one fiber food. Different types of fiber initiate different physiological responses in the human body.

5. Fiber supplements can be taken anywhere (trips, camping etc.).

6. Taking a fiber supplement on a daily basis helps to lower cholesterol levels, speeds transit time, prevents constipation, and contributes to weight management.

TYPES OF FIBER SUPPLEMENTS

BASE	ACTION
Bran Fiber	low solubility with good water holding properties

Psyllium	Colorless transparent mucilage forms around the insoluble seed
Gums	Forms a homogenous adhesive gelatinous mass to expedite colonic waste
Methyl Cellulose	Slowly soluble and creates a viscous, colloid solution
Ispaghula Husk	Swells rapidly to form a mucilage

FIBER SUPPLEMENTS CAN BE ENHANCED BY ADDING:

- herbs such as aloe vera, cascara sagrada, rhubarb, slippery elm or acacia (each of these herbs exerts a tonifying or healing effect on the mucous membranes of the colon).

- calcium, which can help to protect the colon from the development of malignancies.

- GTF chromium enhances insulin utilization and with fiber, contributes to normalizing blood sugar levels which affect food cravings and fat storage.

- vitamins and minerals are also added to some high quality fiber formulas. Obtaining B-vitamins, biotin, vitamin E, ascorbic acid or zinc only enhances the nutritive value of the fiber mix.

Fiber supplements are usually available in powder form and are designed to mix with a liquid. They are typically blended into juices, hot cereals, casseroles, dressings, and gravies. If you find them difficult to take in drink form, think of creative ways to sneak them into moist food like batters (pancake, waffle, cookie, cake etc.), soups or stews.

NOTE: Experience has proven that if you add fiber supplements to your diet, they work better if you rotate them. Popular and effective supplements include: gum acacia, pectin, guar gum, oat fiber, psyllium seed, apple pectin, agar and flaxseed. For optimal results, make sure you get adequate amounts of fiber preparations.

REMEMBER: YOU NEED TO TAKE FIBER SUPPLEMENT FOR AT LEAST THREE MONTHS TO BEGIN TO CONSISTENTLY SEE PHYSIOLOGICAL BENEFITS. BEGIN TO ADD FIBER SLOWLY TO YOUR DIET AND TRY NOT TO OVERDOSE ON JUST ONE TYPE OF FIBER. FIBER FORMULAS THAT INCLUDE A VARIETY OF FIBER OR A MIX OF VITAMINS, HERBS OR MINERALS ARE ESPECIALLY GOOD.

Take your fiber supplement 30 minutes before you eat to help curb your appetite and create satiety and drink plenty of water.

TOTAL FIBER CONTENT OF FIBER SUPPLEMENT SOURCES WITH SOLUBLE AND INSOLUBLE PERCENTAGES*

TYPE OF FIBER	PERCENT SOLUBLE	PERCENT INSOLUBLE	TOTAL
Guar Gum	90.0	0.0	90.0
Pea Fiber	21.0	65.0	90.0
Citrus Pectin	85.8	0.7	86.5
Locust Bean Gum	71.4	11.1	82.5
Soy Fiber	5.2	71.2	76.4
Beet Fiber	24.0	50.5	74.5
Barely Bran	3.0	62.0	65.0
Apple Fiber	1.7	56.0	57.7
Psyllium Husks	47.9	9.7	57.6
Rice Bran	7.7	20.4	28.1
Oat Bran	15.0	3.2	18.2

*Taken from a chart in *New Facts About Fiber* by Betty Kamen, Ph.D.

CONCLUSION:

FIBER IS NOTHING LESS THAN FABULOUS

After studying and learning about fiber and its incredible benefits for human health and well being, I have to admit, I've become somewhat of a fiber fanatic. It is nothing less than remarkable that one natural substance could possess so many health promoting and disease preventing properties. I had no idea.

Let me tell you, my grocery shopping habits will never be the same. I have started to look for fiber content and types on all packaged foods. I use a fiber supplement each and every day and try to drink plenty of pure, unchlorinated water. Wow, I cannot even begin to tell you how differently my colon behaves now! I never suffer from the chronic constipation that has plagued me since I was a child and I feel 100% better in all respects.

One of the most exciting things about eating a fiber-rich diet is that you can actually eat more satisfying food than you did before and NOT gain weight. What a boon to millions of us who used to practically starve ourselves to keep those dreaded pounds from our poor deprived bodies. No more.

I can promise you this much: when you become "fiber aware" you naturally gravitate to whole, raw, fresh foods that are superior in their nutritional content to processed, refined, fiber wimpy, fat-promoting foods. The key is becoming aware and deciding to change. How much evidence does one need. The facts are overwhelming and are nothing less than startling in their health implications.

SIMPLY STATED: SO MANY OF US ARE EITHER SICK OR FAT BECAUSE WE WERE RAISED ON FIBER DEFICIENT DIETS THAT ARE INHERITED BY OUR CHILDREN. LET'S STOP THE CYCLE OF OBESITY AND DISEASE RIGHT NOW.

I have come to believe that making sure that we and our families eat at least 35 grams of fiber per day is probably the one most "healthful" things we can do. I have become such a fiber advocate that I think if I chose to enter politics, I would run on a "fiber" platform. After all, if the entire nation consumed 35 to 40 grams of fiber per day, I believe that the physical, psychological and fiscal ramifications of such a change would be nothing less than astronomical.

REMEMBER OUR NEW CAMPAIGN MOTTO: FIGHT FOR FIBER!

TO SUMMARIZE, THERE ARE FIVE PRIMARY WAYS THAT WE CAN INCREASE OUR DIETARY FIBER:

1. Change to whole meal breads with high fiber contents.

2. Eat breakfast cereals that are high in bran or are made from the whole grain (Oat Bran, Whole Wheat etc.).

3. Dramatically increase the amount of raw fruits and vegetables consumed.

4. Use legumes liberally as substitutes for animal protein or dairy products.

5. Use a high quality extra-dietary fiber supplement daily.

FEAST ON FIBER

THERMOS COOKERY

One of the most convenient and healthful ways to prepare breakfast grains is to use a wide-mouth thermos. The thermos holds in heat and slowly cooks the grain without the kind of high heat that destroys nutrients inherently contained in foods. Thermos cooking heat is well below the boiling point. In essence, the grains cook themselves slowly and gently and in an air-restricted environment. You can place your grains in the thermos, go to bed and wake up to a delicious and nutritious breakfast that is ready to eat!

A wide-mouth thermos is recommended for easy access. Use the following instructions to successfully thermos cook. You'll never go back to cooking cereals in a pot, which can so often result in scorching, sticking and messy boil overs.

1. Purchase a high quality, wide-mouth, glass-lined thermos.
2. Rinse the thermos with scalding water and quickly spoon in the grain.
3. Fill the thermos to the top with boiling water, close tightly and leave to cook overnight or for several hours. Letting the grains cook for 8 to 12 hours is ideal.

NOTE: Use 1/2 cup to 1 1/4 cups of boiling water for a pint-sized thermos. Always pre-wash your grains.

You can use whole wheat, barley, brown rice, buckwheat, milled and whole oats. If you thermos cook millet, you need to bring the grain to the boiling point and simmer it for five minutes prior to putting it in the thermos or the hard, outer husks will not break open.

Louise Tenney combines one cup of each of the following whole grains together: wheat, rye, barley, buckwheat and whole oats. She keeps this mixture on hand for thermos cooking, and before she tightens the lid, adds dates, raisins or figs for natural sweetening. She also grinds almonds or pecans and will add them for a special taste treat.

Thermos cooking is a marvelous way to prepare grain without compromising its nutrient. You don't need a stove or a microwave to thermos cook. It's really just as easy as pulling out a box of Captain Crunch for breakfast and so much better for you.

FIBER-FILLED RECIPES

Louise Tenney, who has written several books on nutrition and herbal medicine, has a marvelous assortment of delicious high-fiber recipes. The following recipes are fiber rich and come from her book, *Today's Healthy Eating*. They have been tried and are most definitely true! Experiment with them and learn to eat healthily again.

FIBER-FUN BREAKFAST DISHES

Grape Nuts

3 C whole wheat flour
1 C sour milk*
1/2 C honey
1/2 C date sugar or brown sugar
1 C ground almonds or pecans
1 tsp sea salt or mineral salt
1 1/2 tsp baking powder
1 Tbsp pure vanilla

*Add 1 tsp apple cider vinegar or lemon juice to milk to make sour milk.

Blend all ingredients in mixer. Place in 12x18 pan. Cook 15 minutes at 350. Cut in squares: turn over. Return to oven. Cook at 200° for 30 minutes. When done, break into little pieces. Put back into oven until crisp and crunchy.

Super Breakfast Cereal

1/2 C oatmeal
1 C plain yogurt
2 T orange juice
1/2 C raisins
1/4 C almonds, chopped
1 T sesame seeds
1/2 C chopped peaches
1/2 C chopped apples
1/2 C sliced bananas

Fold all ingredients together. You can substitute sunflower seeds for sesame seeds or pecans for almonds.

Russian Pancakes

3/4 C of whole wheat (not flour)
1 C milk (almond or soy can also be used)
1/4 tsp sea salt
2 tsp baking powder (aluminum free)
2 eggs (slightly beaten)
1/4 C oil

Combine all ingredients until slightly blended. Pour out on hot griddle. Top with fresh fruit.

Buckwheat Crepes

1/2 C buckwheat flour
1/2 C whole wheat pastry flour
1/4 C wheat germ
1 C milk
1/2 C water
1/2 t mineral salt
3 eggs
3 T cold-pressed oil

Combine flours, eggs, milk, water, salt and oil. Mix in blender. Batter should be thick, but if it is too thick, the crepe will curl up at the edges when cooking. Just add a little more milk. Heat a skillet and spread butter and oil mixture on it, butter alone will burn. Pour 1/3 C of crepe batter on the pan and swirl to cover entire surface or tilt the pan to cover bottom. Cook crepe about one minute and flip over to cook other side. The second side need not be brown for it to be done.

Top with blueberries, strawberries, cherries, peaches, or boysenberries and sour or whipping cream.

Oatmeal Pancakes

1 C whole oat flour
1/4 C oat or wheat bran
3/4 C whole wheat flour
1 T baking powder (aluminum free)
1 t Salt
2 eggs
1 3/4 C milk
1/3 C butter, melted

In a large bowl stir all dry ingredients together. In a smaller bowl, beat the eggs and beat in the milk and butter. Stir this mixture into the dry mixture just until blended. Do not beat, you want the batter to be slightly lumpy. Heat a large skillet which has been brushed with melted butter. Pour 1/4 C batter for each pancake.

Raw Wheat with Fruit

2 T wheat flakes
7 T water
2 T lemon juice
2 T ground sesame seeds
1 T honey or maple syrup
1 small banana
1 t ground almonds
almond milk for moistening

Soak wheat flakes overnight. Mix juice, ground almonds and honey. Dried fruit may be used. Soak overnight, grind and add to any cereal.

Raw Granola

6 C raw oatmeal (baby oat)
1 C ground sunflower seed
1 C ground sesame seeds
1/4 C ground chia seeds
1 C ground flaxseeds
1 C shredded coconut
1 C ground almonds
1 1/2 t grated orange rind
1/2 t cardamom
1 C date sugar
1/2 C warm honey

Mix all dry ingredients together and then drip the warm honey on the mixture and stir. Spread on a greased cookie sheet and cook in the oven at 200° for about an hour, stirring often. Store in a tight jar in a cool place or freeze.

NOTE: This granola is a great intestinal "broom" and helps to sweep unwanted waste from the colon.

Fruit and Seeds

1/4 C ground sunflower seeds
1/4 C ground sesame seeds
1/2 C white figs or dates
1/2 C spring water

Soak seeds and dry fruit overnight in spring water. Blend all ingredients in a blender. Pour over fresh apples, bananas or peaches. Makes a quick and nourishing breakfast.

Orange Corn-Bran Muffins

1 1/4 C all-purpose flour
3/4 C corn bran
1/2 C cornmeal
2 tsp baking powder
1 tsp baking soda
1/2 tsp salt
3/4 C buttermilk
1/2 C orange juice
1/3 C dark brown sugar, firmly packed
1/4 C canola oil
2 egg whites
2 tsp grated orange rind
1/2 tsp vanilla extract

Preheat oven to 400°. Grease 12 muffin cups. In a large bowl, stir together the flour, corn bran, cornmeal, baking powder, baking soda and salt. In a medium size bowl, stir together the buttermilk, orange juice, brown sugar, oil, egg whites, orange rind and vanilla. Add the orange mixture to the dry ingredients and stir until just moistened. Spoon into prepared cups and bake 20 minutes.

Soups

Bean Soup

1 C any type of beans
4 C pure water
1 C grated carrots
1 small onion, grated
1/2 C parsley, chopped
1 T nut cream
1 t lemon juice

Soak beans overnight in three cups of water. Cook beans in 4 cups of water until tender. Blend the cooked beans and vegetables in a blender, add parsley, nut cream and lemon and let boil for a few minutes.

Chili Corn Soup

3 T oil
1 Onion, chopped
1 green pepper, chopped
1 clove of garlic, minced
3 stalks of celery, chopped
1 Qt. of stewed tomatoes
1 T chili powder
1 t oregano
1 t basil
2 C fresh or frozen corn
2 C cooked pinto or red beans
2 C vegetable broth

Saute oil with onion, pepper, garlic and celery. Cook until transparent. Add tomatoes, broth, spices and cook for 30 minutes. Add all other ingredients and cook for 20 more minutes.

Split Pea Soup

1 C dried split peas
4 C pure cold water
1 medium onion, minced
1 C celery chopped
2 small carrots, grated
2 T chopped parsley
1/2 C nut cream
1 t sea salt

Soak the peas overnight and cook in the same water for about two hours. When done, add the nut cream and seasoning.

Lentil Soup

2 C lentils
5 C bran water
1 quart stewed tomatoes
2 stalks celery, chopped
1 large green pepper
2 large carrots, chopped
2 cloves garlic, minced
1/2 t basil
1/4 C tamari
salt to taste

Combine all ingredients except kelp in a slow cooker. Cover and cook on low heat for about 6 hours. Season to taste.

Okra and Barley Soup

1/2 pound of okra, frozen or fresh
1 small onion
1 T arrowroot
1/2 C barley, cooked
3 C nut milk

Steam the chopped okra and onion until tender. Mix arrowroot with nut milk and cook slowly in a double boiler with okra, onion and cooked barley, until done.

Everything Vegetable Soup

1/2 C dried pinto beans
1/2 C dried garbanzo beans
1/2 C dried Great Northern Beans
2 C vegetable broth
1 T salt
1 t ground cumin
1 t chili powder
2 C mild vegetable juice
2 C tomato juice
2 lbs fresh tomatoes
1/2 C dried lima beans
1 C uncooked brown rice
3 medium onions, diced
3 medium carrots, sliced
3 stalks of celery, sliced
3 medium unpeeled potatoes, diced
2 C whole kernel corn
2 C water

Combine the first 9 ingredients in a 5-quart pot or dutch oven and bring to a boil. Reduce the heat to simmer covered for 1 hour. Remove the stem ends from the tomatoes, cut them into chunks and put them once through the blender. Add the tomatoes, dried limas and brown rice to the mixture in the pot. Bring to a boil, reduce heat and simmer covered until the limas and rice are almost tender. Add the remaining ingredients and continue to simmer until the carrots are tender. This soup is thick and resembles a stew. If you like yours a bit thinner, add more liquid. Serves 8 to 10 people.

MEATLESS MAIN DISHES

Zucchini and Oat Groats

Any variety of squash can be used for this dish.

2 T of canola or olive oil
1/2 C chopped onion
1/2 C chopped parsley
2 C of chopped squash
1 C oat groats
1 can of chicken broth
1 clove of garlic, minced
salt to taste

Heat the oil in a two quart sauce pan and saute the onion and garlic until the onion is transparent and soft. Add the broth and bring to a boil, Blend in the oats and simmer for 30 minutes. Stir in the squash, parsley and salt. Cover and cook on low for 10 minutes more.

MULTI-GRAIN STEW

1/2 C whole rye
1/2 C whole wheat berries
1/2 C barley
1/2 C millet
8 C water
1 large onion, chopped
2 stalks of celery, diced
2 leeks, sliced
1 large sweet potato, coarsely chopped
1 clove garlic, minced
1 (16oz.) can tomatoes, chopped with liquid
1/2 C chopped fresh parsley
2 T soy sauce
1 t paprika
1 t basil
1/2 t ground cumin
1/4 t white pepper
1/2 t hot pepper sauce
1 can green chilies

Place all ingredients in a large pot. Bring to a boil, reduce heat, cover and simmer for 3 hours (in a slow cooker, cook 8 hours on high). Stir occasionally. Serves eight. Four whole grains are featured in this good-tasting and satisfying stew.

BAKED RICE AND MILLET

1 1/2 C cooked brown rice
1/2 C cooked milled
2 eggs beaten
2 C. milk
2 T butter
1 T tamari soy sauce
1 C chopped almonds
1/4 C chopped sunflower seeds

Mix all ingredients. Pour into a 2 quart casserole dish. Bake at 30 minutes at 350° degrees.

BEAN BURGERS

2 C pinto beans, cooked
1 C brown rice, cooked
2 eggs
2 cloves garlic, pressed
1/4 C wheat germ
1/4 C sunflower seeds, ground
1/4 C almonds, ground
2 T what bran
Season wheat bran with vegetable salt, kelp or miso

Mix all ingredients together. Roll patties in wheat bran. Fry in a small amount of olive oil.

BEAN AND MILLET SUPPER

1 C pinto beans, cooked
1 C milled, cooked
1/4 C almonds, ground
3 T butter
1 C onions, chopped
1 C mushrooms, chopped
1/2 C green peepers, chopped
1/2 C celery, chopped
1 t vegetable broth seasoning
3 t lemon juice
1/8 t rosemary
1/8 t sage

Saute the onions, peppers, mushrooms and celery with butter. Add seasonings and lemon juice with 1/2 C water. Cook on low for about 10 minutes. Add beans, millet and almonds. Serves 4.

CHILI BEANS

1 C dried pinto beans
2 C water
1 T olive oil
1 large onion, chopped
1 clove garlic, minced
1 green pepper, minced
1 qt canned tomatoes
1 t chili powder
1 t paprika
1 t blackstrap molasses
1/2 t cumin

Pre-soak beans overnight. Throw away the soaking water. Add boiling eater to cover and cook for at least 30 minutes. Discard the cooking water (this helps to get rid of the trisaccharides that can cause gas).

Add fresh water (about 2 cups or more) and resume cooking until done. Add remaining ingredients and continue to cook for about 1 hour.

GARBANZO STEW

1 qt of canned tomatoes
1 qt pure water
1 C garbanzo beans
1 C carrots
1 C potatoes with skin on
1/4 C millet
1 t mineral salt
1 T vegetable powder

Soak garbanzo beans overnight in 2 cups of water. Cook beans in tomatoes in one qt. of water. Cook until tender. Add millet and cook thirty minutes. Add chopped carrots, diced potatoes, salt and vegetable powder. Cook until tender.

POTATO SUPREME

Bake 1 potato for each person

In a saucepan, saute, 2 cups mushrooms in 4 T butter with one clove of minced garlic. Simmer lightly, and don't let the mushrooms get soggy. Open up potatoes. Put in butter, grated cheese, sour cream, chopped black olives, and chopped chives. Top with sauteed, mushrooms. Use your imagination for baked potatoes with chili, stroganoff etc.

STUFFED PEPPERS

6 large green peppers
2 T butter or ghee
4 small onions
1 C cooked brown rice
1 C cooked millet
1 C almonds, ground fine
1 C grated cheese
4 eggs, beaten
salt and pepper to taste

Remove the pulp and seeds of the peppers. Saute onions in butter. Mix all other ingredients with the onions and butter. Stuff each pepper until full. Arrange the peppers open end up in a baking dish. Pour water into the dish to barely cover the bottom. Bake for 30 minutes at 350°. Leftover stuffing can be used for a casserole.

STUFFED PUMPKIN

2-4 lb pumpkin or acorn squash
2 C brown rice (cooked)
1 C wild rice (cooked)
2 C whole wheat bread crumbs
1 large onion, chopped
1 C chopped celery with tops
1 C green apples, chopped
1 C ground walnuts
1 t poultry seasoning
1 1/2 t vegetable broth
1/2 C butter or canola oil
soy sauce or salt and pepper to taste

Combine all ingredients. Saute onions and celery in butter or oil and mix well. Add soy or salt. Add all ingredients together. The stuffing should be moist. If you like a drier stuffing, use less liquid. Cut the top off the pumpkin. Remove the seeds and any stringy pulp. Pack the stuffing loosely in the pumpkin. Put the lid on the pumpkin and bake on an oiled baking sheet for about 1 1/2 hours at 325°. When you serve the stuffed pumpkin, scoop out the pumpkin along with the stuffing.

PASTA FAGGIOLI (BEANS) PESTO

1/4 C pine nuts (shelled)
1/4 C olive oil
1/2 C fresh basil or 1 t dried basil
3 cloves of minced garlic
2 C whole grain pasta
2 C cooked or canned white beans
1/2 C grated Parmesan
1 t butter

Cook the pine nuts in a dry frying pan until brown. Take off the heat. Add oil, basil, and garlic to a blender or food processor and blend until the basil is finely chopped. Cook the pasta according to directions. Drain and toss with butter. Add the beans and the pesto sauce and re-heat. Top with parmesan cheese.

BREADS, MUFFINS AND CRACKERS

GRAHAM CRACKERS

2 C whole wheat graham flour
1 C whole wheat pastry flour
1/2 C ground sesame seeds
2 T arrowroot
1/2 C cold pressed oil
1/2 C water
1/2 C molasses

Work the oil into all the dry ingredients. Mix the water and the molasses together and blend into dry mixture. Knead the dough and roll our thin. Cut into squares and prick with a fork. Bake at 300° for 25 minutes.

MILLET CRACKERS

1 T dried yeast
1/2 C lukewarm water
1/2 C hot water
1/2 C dried apricots
1/2 C dried light figs
1 C cold pressed oil
3 C millet flour
1 C whole wheat flour

Pour the yeast in the lukewarm water. Pour the hot water in a blender and add the apricots and figs and blend into fine meal. Combine yeast and fruit together. Stir in the oil and the flours. The dough should be stiff. Add more flour if you need to. Roll out on floured board and cut into squares. Place on oiled cooked sheet and let stand 15 minutes before baking at 300° for about 30 minutes.

APPLE/RAISIN MUFFINS

1 C whole-wheat flour
1 C unbleached white flour
2 T maple sugar
2 t baking powder
1/2 t baking soda (aluminum free)
1/2 t salt
1/2 t all spice
1 C of vanilla yogurt
2 T canola oil
1/2 C applesauce
1 egg
2 apples, peeled and chopped
1/2 C raisins
1/2 C walnuts

Coat inside of muffin pan with non-stick spray. In a large bowl, combine all dry ingredients. Fold in the moist ingredients and the egg and blend but do not beat. Add the raisins and the walnuts and bake at 400° for 20 minutes.

BRAN MUFFINS

1 C bran
1 1/2 C whole wheat pastry flour
1 1/4 t baking powder (aluminum free)
1 beaten egg
3/4 C milk
1/4 C honey
2 T cold pressed oil
1 t orange rind

Mix all ingredients together. Spoon batter into greased muffin tins. Bakes for 20 minutes at 400° or until muffins begin to pull away from pan. Makes a dozen. For a special treat add a cup of grated fresh apples to batter.

ALMOND-SUNFLOWER SEED MUFFINS

1 C ground sunflower seeds
1 C ground almonds
1/4 C sesame seeds
1/2 C wheat germ
1/2 C rice polishings
1/2 C unsweetened coconut

Combine dry ingredients. Add the following ingredients and fold the egg whites in last.

3 egg yolks
2 T honey
2 1/2 T cold pressed oil
1 C orange juice
3 beaten egg whites

Fill grease muffin tins 3/4 full and bake at 350° for about 25 minutes.

BLUEBERRY MUFFINS

1 3/4 C whole wheat pastry flour
1/4 C wheat germ
4 t baking powder (aluminum free)
1/2 t pure vanilla
1 t salt
1 egg
6 T cold pressed oil
1/4 C honey
1 T lecithin
1 C sesame milk
1 C blueberries (fresh or frozen)

Blend all the dry ingredients together. Beat egg, oil, honey and lecithin together and stir into dry mixture. Add milk and fold in blueberries, Put in greased muffin tins and bake at 375° for 25 minutes.

NO FAIL WHOLE WHEAT BREAD

Dissolve 4 T dry yeast into a mix of 1/2 C honey or molasses and 6 C warm water. Add 2 T sea salt and 8 C of whole wheat flour and blend well. Beat at least 100 times or use a bread mixer. Let stand for 20 minutes. Add 10 T cold pressed oil, 1 C bran, 1 C wheat germ and 6 more cups of flour. Knead. Cover and let rise for 30 minutes till double in bulk. Form into 4 loaves, place in greased loaf pans and let rise for 30 more minutes. Bake at 350° for 45 minutes to 1 hour.

A GLOSSARY
OF GRAINS

Amaranth: Considered the sacred grain of the Aztec Indians, it was cultivated for almost 8,000 years before its disappearance in the early 1500s. Recently, it has been revived and is currently used in a number of American recipes. It is a source of total amino acid nutrition, which unlike some grains, makes it a complete protein. It is routinely toasted, popped or mixed in with other whole grains or milled into flour.

Barley: This particular grain has a low fiber content but contains a whole host of desirable nutrients. It is considered an ancient cereal and was routinely used by the Egyptian culture. Because it is so easy to digest, it is recommended for anyone who is allergic to other grains. It makes a wonderful addition to soups and stews.

Blue Corn: This variety of corn is richer in nutrients than- yellow corn and is higher in protein content and complex carbohydrates. The Hopi Indians used it to sustain the body under periods of high physical stress. It is rich in iron, zinc, magnesium, phosphorus, copper and potassium.

Brown Rice: Brown rice is considered a panacea among whole grains. It is a whole, unpolished grain which retains its bran and germ intact. Because of its superior balance of nutrients, it is regarded as a marvelous food. Eating brown rice provides a rich supply of B-complex vitamins. It feeds over 50% of the world's population and has been used therapeutically for a number of disorders.

Buckwheat: A food that has provided nourishment for human beings since 8000 B.C., buckwheat can be considered a fruit and is a distant cousin to rhubarb. When buckwheat is dried, it reveals a pale kernel called a groat. Buckwheat is high is B-vitamins, protein and is an excellent source of complex carbohydrates. Buckwheat can be used in muffins, pancakes and casseroles. It is lower in calories than wheat, rice or corn and richer in protein.

Corn: Corn and corn by-products essentially replaced wheat decades ago. Some experts believe that the glut of corn-related foods has diminished the quality of our health, Degerminated cornmeal is basically fiberless and bolted cornmeal contains the germ but not the corn bran. Corn bran can be a good source of fiber.

Couscous: Relatively unknown, couscous is nothing more than a type of pasta made from semolina wheat. It is a favorite in France and has seen limited success here as an addition to side dishes.

Kamut: A relatively large kernel grain, kamut is a rich source of protein and contains more lipids and minerals than wheat.

Millet: Millet is the micrograin of grains. It resembles birdseed and has a long history of use. Its high protein content makes it a good addition to foods. Using millet in stuffings, soups and stews is gaining popularity.

Oats: Oats have truly experience a renaissance over the last few years. The ability of oat bran to lower cholesterol levels resulted in a veritable oat frenzy. Unquestionably, oats provide good nutrition and oat bran is an excellent source of fiber.

Rye: Rye is a hearty and flavorful grain that is considered a staple in Russia and parts of Eastern Europe. It is typically mixed with other grains.

Quinoa: Like, amaranth, quinoa is a complete protein which was also used by ancient South American Indians and called the mother grain by Chileans. It is considered a perfect food in that it contains a complete array of nutrients. Sometimes categorized as a fruit, quinoa is experiencing renewed interest today.

Spelt: Spelt was cultivated in parts of Europe and is considered one of the earliest grains used by man. It is higher in protein, fats and fiber than wheat and is a good substitute for anyone who has a food intolerance to wheat.

Teff: Used by the Greeks and Ethiopians, Teff is also higher in some nutrients than wheat.

Triticale: Several years ago triticale almost became a household word in that it received considerable media attention. It exceeds the protein content of wheat and has a superior blend of amino acids. It can be purchased in ground or flake form and is basically a combination of wheat and rye.

Wheat: Wheat has been the primary choice of grains for human beings since pre-historic times. Wheat germ, wheat bran and wheat berries have all recently emerged as highly nutritive extracts of whole wheat. Wheat is clearly the most popular grain worldwide. Recent emphasis on consuming wheat in its whole form has resulted in a dramatic increase of whole wheat bread and other products.

Wild Rice: Considered a gourmet side dish, wild rice is exclusively native to North America. Very much unlike other varieties of rice, it has been used by Native Americans and is relatively expensive.

ENDNOTES

[1] T.A. Nicklas, R.P. Farris, L. Meyers, G.S. Berensen, *Journal of the American Dietetic Association.* (Feb. 1995, 95(2): 209-14.

[2] Mark L. Dreher, *Handbook of Dietary Fiber.* (New York: Marcel Dekker, INC., 1987), 6.

[3] Ibid.

[4] David Kritchevsky, Charles Bonfield and James W. Anderson, eds., *Dietary Fiber.* (New York and London: Plenum Press, 1988), XII.

[5] Dreher, 11.

[6] Alma E. Guiness, ed., *Family Guide to Natural Medicine.* (Pleasantville, New York: The Reader's Digest Association Inc., 1993.) 254, from "Laurel's Kitchen" by Laurel Robertson, Carol Flinders and Bronwen Godfrey.

[7] Michael Murray N.D. and Joseph Pizzorno N.D., *Encyclopedia of Natural Medicine.* (Rocklin, California: Prima Publishing, 1991), 41.

[8] Leon Prosky and Jonathan Devries, *Controlling Dietary Fiber in Food Products.* (New York: Van Nostrand Reinhold, 1992), 12.

[9] A.M. Stephen, "Whole Grains—impact of consuming whole grains on physiological effects of dietary fiber and starch," *Critical Review, Food Science and Nutrition.* (1994; 34(5-6): 499-511.

[10] David Kritchevsky and Charles Bonfield, *Dietary Fiber in Health and Disease.* (St. Paul, Minnesota: Eagan Press, 1995), 8.

[11] Prosky, 17.

[12] Anne Fletcher, M.S., R.D. "Food and Your Health, The Facts on Fiber."

[13] Zecharia Madar, and H. Selwyn Odes, *Dietary Fiber Research.* (Switzerland: Thur AG Offsetdruck,

Pratteln, 1990), 67.

[14] Louise Tenney, *Encyclopedia of Natural Remedies.* (Pleasant Grove, Utah: Woodland Publishing, 1995), 177.

[15] G.W. Neal and T.K. Balm, "Synergistic effects of psyllium in the dietary treatment of hypercholesterolemia," *Southern Medical Journal,* Oct. 1990: 83(10): 1131-7.

[16] Brian K Bailey, D.P.M., and Susan Smith Jones, Ph.D. "Ten Ways to Increase Your Metabolism," *Let's Live,* 8: 1994.

[17] B. McNamee, and V. Mansour-McNamee, *Dietary Fiber,* (Baltimore: Urban and Schwarzenberg, 1989), 24.

[18] Hoover-Plow, J., J. Savesky and G. Dailey, "The glycemic response to meals with six different fruits in insulin-dependent diabetes using a home blood-glucose monitoring system," *American Journal of Clinical Nutrition,* Jan. 1987: 45(1): 92-7.

[19] T. Poynard et al., "Reduction of post-prandial insulin needs by pectin as assessed by the artificial pancreas in insulin-dependent diabetics," *Diabetes and Metabolism* 1982: 8(3): 187-9.

[20] S.J. Fairweather-Tait and A.J. Wright, "The effect of sugar-beet fibre and wheat bran on iron and zinc absorption in rats," *British Journal of Nutrition,* Sept. 1990: 64(2): 547-52.

[21] McNamee, 63.

[22] Kritchevsky, *Dietary Fiber in Health and Disease,* 264.

[23] Hugh Trowell, Denis Burkitt, and Kenneth Heaton, *Dietary Fibre, Fibre-Depleted Foods and Disease,* (London: Academic Press, 1985), 200.

[24] Ibid., 198.

[25] Ibid., 199.

[26] Jon J. Michnovicz, M.D., Ph.D., *How to Reduce Your Risk of Breast Cancer,* (New York: Warner Books, 1994), 7.

[27] Charles B. Clayman, M.D. ed., *Home Medical Encyclopedia,* The American Medical Association, (New York: Random House, 1989), 206.

[28] Kritchevsky, *Dietary Fiber in Health and Disease,* 166.

[29] Ibid.

[30] Ibid., 167.

[31] Michnovicz, 115.

[32] Ibid.

[33] Trowell, 225.

[34] Ibid.

[35] S. Leo et al., "Ulcerative colitis in remission: is it possible to predict the risk of relapse?" *Digestion,* 1989: 44(4): 217-21.

[36] Sid Kirchheimer, *The Doctor's Book of Home Remedies,* (Emmaus, Pennsylvania: Rodale Press, 1993), 121.

[37] J. Snook and H.A. Shepherd, "Bran supplementation in the treatment of irritable bowel syndrome," *Ailment-Pharmacology-Therapeutics* Oct. 1994: 8(5): 511-4.

[38] Dreher, 287.

[39] Richard A. Passwater, Ph.D., *Cancer Prevention and Nutritional Therapies,* (New Canaan, Connecticut: Keats Publishing, 1993), 153.

[40] Ibid.

[41] Ibid., 154.

[42] Ibid., 156.

[43] U.S. Department of Health and Human Services, *Healthy People 2000: National Health Promotion and Disease Prevention Objectives.* (Washington, D.C.: DHHS Publication, 1991), No. (PHS) 91-50213.

[44] Dreher, 297.

[45] T.F. Schweizer and C. A. Edwards, eds., *Dietary Fibre, A Component of Food, Nutritional Function in Health and Disease,* (London: Springer-Verlag, 1992),

322.

[46] Kritchevsky, *Dietary Fiber in Health and Disease,* 140.

[47] J.A. Story, "Dietary Fiber and lipid metabolism," *Medical Aspects of Dietary Fiber,* (New York: Plenum Medical, 1980), 138.

[48] H. Lipsky, M. Gloger and W.H. Frishman, "Dietary Fiber for reducing blood cholesterol, *Journal of Clinical Pharmacology,* Aug. 1990: 30(8): 699- 703.

[49] B.P. Kinosian and J.M. Eisenber, "Cutting into cholesterol. Cost-effective alternatives for treating hypercholesterolemia," *Journal of the American Medical Association,* April 15, 1988: 259(15): 2249-54.

[50] D. Kromhout, "Dietary fiber and 10-year mortality for coronary heart disease, cancer and all causes," *Lancet* 1982: 2: 518-22.

[51] Kritchevsky, *Dietary Fiber in Health and Disease,* 132.

[52] Trowell, 264.

[53] Ibid.

[54] Ibid., 268.

[55] Ibid., 270.

[56] McNamee, 35

[57] Ibid., 36.

[58] Trowell, 271.

[59] D.A. Jenkins et al. "Treatment of Diabetes with guar gum: Reduction of urinary glucose loss in diabetics," *Lancet* 1977: 2:779.

[60] Trowell, 269.

[61] J.W. Anderson and K. Ward, "High-carbohydrate, high-fiber diets for insulin-treated men with diabetes mellitus," *American Journal of Clinical Nutrition,* 1979: 32: 2312-21.

[62] McNamee, 41.

[63] Trowell, 151.

[64] Ibid., 155.

[65] Ibid.

[66] Ibid., 155.

[67] B. J. Smits, A.M. Whitehead and P. Prescott, "Lactulose in the treatment of symptomatic diverticular disease: a comparative study with high-fibre diet," *British Journal of Clinical Practice* Aug. 1990: 44(8): 314.

[68] James Scala, M.D., *Eating Right for a Bad Gut,* (New York: Penguin Books, 1990), 123.

[69] Trowell, 156.

[70] Ibid., 290.

[71] Dreher, 303.

[72] G.G. Birch and K. J. Parker, *Dietary Fiber,* (London: Applied Science Publishers, 1983), 199.

[73] H. Andersson et al. *Human Nutrition: Applied Nutrition,* Apr. 1985: 39A: 101.

[74] Trowell, 247.

[75] Ibid., 242.

[76] Ibid.

[77] D.P. Burkitt et. al. *Lancet,* Oct. 1985: 2:880.

[78] Trowell, 246.

[79] Schweizer, 274.

[80] Ibid.

[81] P. Little et al., "A controlled trial of low sodium, low fat, high fiber diet in treated hypersensitive patients: the efficacy of multiple dietary intervention," *Postgraduate Medical Journal* Aug. 1990: 66(778): 616-21.

[82] G. J. Keitch et al., "Dietary fiber and giardiasis: dietary fiber reduces rate of intestinal infection by Giardia lamblia in the gerbil," *American Journal of Tropical Medicine and Hygiene,* Nov. 1989: 41(5): 512-520.

[83] A. Rydning et al., "Prophylactic effect of dietary fiber in duodenal ulcer disease," *Lancet,* 1982: 2:736.

[84] Kritchevsky, *Dietary Fiber in Health and Disease,* 193.

[85] Trowell, 320.

[86] Ibid., 321.

[87] *Forbes Magazine,* December 5, 1994.

[88] Kritchevsky, *Dietary Fiber in Health and Disease,* 378.

[89] *Let's Live,* August, 1994.

[90] Daniel B. Mowrey, Ph.D. *The Scientific Validation of Herbal Medicine,* (New Canaan, Connecticut: Keats Publishing, 1986), 278.

QUIZ ANSWERS

The correct answer to each and every statement was false! Let's go through them individually.

1. **FALSE:** Bran is one type of fiber that comprises the outer covering of whole wheat and whole oats. When you buy unprocessed bran, you are getting grain hulls that would normally be discarded when whole wheat or oats are milled. The technical definition of fiber is the residue derived from plant foods that is resistant to human digestive enzymes or also known as "unavailable carbohydrates." The plant cell wall contains structural materials called cellulose and non-cellulose fibers and non-structural polysaccharides.

2. **FALSE:** There are many different kinds of fiber and each has its own particular physiological benefit. For example, wheat bran is wonderful for its bulking abilities. Other forms of fiber such as oat bran are better for cholesterol level lowering etc. For this reason, its important that we eat a variety of fibery foods and take a good fiber supplement to complement our diets.

3. **FALSE:** Beef has no fiber at all. While meat might look "fibrous," it contains no fiber. Fiber comes from vegetable, fruit or grain sources.

4. **FALSE:** When you juice an apple, your juicer will usually discard the peeling and the pulp. These are the fiber-rich parts that contribute to the slower assimilation of sugar when you eat a whole apple. This is why any weight loss diet will usually always

recommend that you eat a whole apple, orange, grapes etc. rather than to drink its juice. It also takes several fruits to provide a full glass of juice, so caloric content and sugar ingestion is much higher in juices. To make matters worse, the fiber is missing from juice, which helps to control the way those calories are metabolized.

5. **FALSE:** Most of the time, cooking or altering whole foods will degrade their fiber content. Potatoes however need cooking to release fiber (so this answer is only partially false).

6. **FALSE:** While supplementing your diet with bran products or grain by-products can be desirable, eating foods in their whole, unaltered state is always better. When you eat the whole grain, with its wheat germ intact and its natural bran covering, your body processes all parts of the grain together. The synergistic effects of that kind of digestion and assimilation are optimal.

7. **FALSE:** Four raw carrot sticks have almost 2 grams of dietary fiber as opposed to the 4 grams found in a small potato.

8. **FALSE:** Cream of Wheat has 3.1 grams of total dietary fiber and Lucky Charms has 4.3. We're talking fiber here, not sugar. Lucky Charms are not recommended as a breakfast food regardless of the fact that they beat out Cream of Wheat in total fiber content.

9. **FALSE:** This is a common notion and is based on the idea that too much fiber might keep essential vitamins and minerals from being absorbed. Cultures

which routinely eat much higher fiber contents than we would ever think of eating do not show nutrient deficiencies. Most of us are fiber depleted. Becoming nutrient deficient because we increase our fiber is not a very credible likelihood.

10. **FALSE:** Even if you are drinking the same amount of apples as opposed to eating them in whole form, their fiber content is missing. Therefore, the body assimilates apple sugar in a different way than if its fiber "buffer" were present. In other worlds, the presence of the fiber in fruit keeps insulin levels under control, helping to normalize blood sugar which is intrinsically related to food cravings and fat storage. Eat the whole apple and skip the juice.

11. **FALSE:** Dr. Burkitt believed that fiber was undigestible and while that is true of some insoluble fibers, some digestive activity takes place. Fibers like bran remain, for the most part, undigested in the large intestine which is why they are so beneficial. This roughage helps to "sweep" the colon clean and keep thing moving right along.

12. **FALSE:** Whether it be fortified 12 ways or 20, eating bread that has been made from ground whole wheat flour is always preferable to refined, bleached white bread. Artificially adding vitamins and minerals which have been stripped away by the milling process can never take the place of Mother Nature's original food. When you eat bread with natural bran and wheat germ, you get the benefit of the whole food and all of its complex, interrelated biochemical reactions.

13. **FALSE:** To the contrary, lettuce and tomatoes are

low fiber foods and while they have their place in our diets, do little for our colonic health. A tossed green salad needs to be fiber fortified with broccoli, pumpkin seeds, beets, carrots, garbanzo beans, red beans etc. to be fiber acceptable.

14. **FALSE, FALSE, FALSE:** This is one of the most widespread fallacies that so many of us fall prey to. According to food charts and RDA requirements, we could be eating white bread, lettuce, cold cereals, custards, ice cream etc. and believe that our overall tally of nutrition was adequate. Sadly, fiber is usually left out of this equation. To get current recommended requirements of fiber, most of us need to re-think how we eat, make adjustments, and even add fiber supplements.

15. **FALSE:** Whether flour is bleached or unbleached has little to do with its fiber content. Remember one of our mottos, "Just because it's brown doesn't mean its fiber rich." Terms to look for are "stone ground" which does not remove fiber and nutrients from the grain and "whole grain."

Score Evaluations:

15-10 points: FIBER GENIUS
9-5 points: FIBER AVERAGE
4-0 points: FIBER FLUNKIE

Index